7 STEPS TO DENTAL HEALTH

I wish you well in your pursuit of holistic health.

Life Learning Series # 3
The Life Transformation Institute

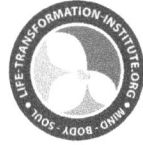

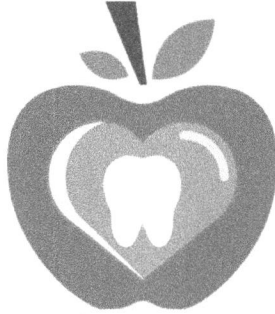

STEPS TO
DENTAL HEALTH

A Holistic Guide to a Healthy Mouth and Body

Avoid Expensive Dental Costs and Live a Healthy Life

THIRD EDITION

Max Haroon
with Dr. Oksana Sawiak and Klaus Ferlow

Contributors
Dr. Brian Clement
Dr. Dana Colson
Dr. Eric Grief
Dr. Iris Kivity-Chandler
Dr. Michael Schecter
Dr. Brian McLean
Dr. Hans-Jurgen Schwartz

Title
7 Steps to Dental Health

Subtitles
A Holistic Guide to a Healthy Mouth and Body
Avoid Expensive Dental Costs and Live a Healthy Life

Author
Max Haroon

Co-authors
Dr. Oksana Sawiak, Klaus Ferlow

Cover Design
Vaughn Dragland, Eclipse Technologies Inc.

Publisher
Life Transformation Institute http://life-transformation-institute.org/.
This book is third in the series "Life Learning".

Book Website
http://www.7stepsdentalhealth.com/

ISBN-13
978-0987882806 (Paperback)
978-0987882820 (eReader) 978-0987882813 (PDF)

ISBN-10
0987882805 (Paperback)

Library and Archives Canada Cataloguing in Publication
Haroon, Max, 1942-, author
7 steps to dental health: a holistic guide to a healthy mouth and body
/ Max Haroon with Dr. Oksana Sawiak and Klaus Ferlow.

(Life learning series; #3)
"Avoid expensive medical costs and live a healthy life."
Includes bibliographical references.
Issued in print and electronic formats.
ISBN 978-0-9878828-0-6 (pbk.).--ISBN 978-0-9878828-1-3 (html)

1. Teeth--Care and hygiene. 2. Mouth--Care and hygiene. 3. Dental care. 4. Nutrition and dental health. 5. Health. I. Sawiak, Oksana, author II. Ferlow, Klaus, author III. Life Transformation Institute IV. Title. V. Title: Seven steps to dental health.

RK61.H37 2014   617.6'01   C2013-908185-2
                                          C2013-908186-0

DISCLAIMER

Every effort has been made to make this book as complete and as accurate as possible. However, there may be mistakes, both typographical and in content.

Authors, Contributors, and the Life Transformation Institute shall have neither liability nor responsibility to any person or entity with respect to any loss or damage caused, or alleged to have been caused, directly or indirectly, by the information contained in this book.

The opinions, recommendations and information provided by all contributors are not necessarily subscribed to by the Life Transformation Institute. The views and opinions expressed by the authors are their own. Products and services mentioned are not endorsed by the Life Transformation Institute or the authors. Neither the Life Transformation Institute nor the authors are linked with any businesses mentioned in the book.

The information is intended as a general guide and not intended as medical advice and we disclaim any liability resulting from its use. It is strongly advocated that each reader seek advice of a qualified professional for medical problems, including those involving dental health.

IN PRAISE OF THIS BOOK

Max Haroon has taken a difficult topic like dental care and transformed it into an easy seven-step process that anyone can do. He has recruited natural health experts in the field to add their vast professional expertise.

Dr. Eric Grief, MD, CCFP.
Bramalea Health Center, Ontario. Author,
Get Diagnosed Fast

Seven Steps to Dental Health by Max Haroon is an amazing and comprehensive book on the dental health. It talks about the bigger picture of how the mouth and body connects. It has a lot of information about the interconnections at many different levels - nutrition to oral hygiene, dental products to wellness. I commend him on his seriousness to tell people how to look after their health starting from their teeth.

Dr. Dana G. Colson, DDS.
Author, Your Mouth: The Gateway to a Healthier You

Max Haroon has dedicated over 3 years into researching and collaborating for this book. One can see that the comprehensive text and related photos can enhance anyone's knowledge in both their dental and overall health. There is undisputed evidence that the health of the mouth is reflective of one's total health. Here in 7 Steps to Dental Health there is detailed information in both integrative and conventional healthcare that will certainly reverse and prevent difficult and costly treatments. For many Holistic practitioners, and certainly for myself, conventional pharmacology-based treatments of TMD, Headaches, Craniofacial Pain and other ailments has given way to an integrative and natural approach that is achieving great results. I will not hesitate to share the knowledge from this book with those under my care and other colleagues who want to empower themselves and their patients.

Dr. Iris Kivity-Chandler, DDS, Cert.
Ortho, M. Sc. Toronto, Orthodontics, TMD and Craniofacial pain

This is the first book I have seen which can help people maintain healthy teeth and gums the totally natural way, so they can avoid dentists whose interventions can often make matters much worse.

Louise McLean. Homeopathic Practitioner, London, UK

Just a few pages into "7 Steps to Holistic Dental Health", it grabbed me. It turned out to be a real "page-turner"; made me want to keep reading like a suspense-thriller! And why not? The level of "intrigue" and "villainy" at play is epic; and, like a prize-winning documentary, the information is presented such that the impact on the reader's life pulls them deeper into the tragic reality of the story being told. Sure, it walks the delicate line between being educated and alarmist, but ultimately, that interpretation comes down to the state of consciousness of the reader.

Attila Lendvai, MBA. Author 'Atlas Project'

I have been told many times to 'tell it like a story' when describing a product. Well, it is not hard to do with this new book 7 Steps to Dental Health. I have been a practicing Dental Hygienist for about 22 years; my excitement for this book cannot be contained. The way that Max Haroon has taken the time to network facts, ask for knowledge and keep on asking is without doubt scientific and trusted reading material. My goal is to help spread the good news that there is now a Holistic Dental Bible.

Victoria DaCosta, RDH, BSDH, SHC.
Systemic Hygiene Consultant, USA

"Maintaining oral balance must be done in conjunction with overall balance. Unfortunately, achieving balance and health can be a confusing and a complicated task. There is a lack of credible information available. The book 7 Steps to Dental Health is a useful, comprehensive read detailing a path of health and success."

Dr Michael Schecter, Schecter Dental Practice, Toronto

Seven Steps to Dental Health, is a great gift to everyone's health. Although a daily affair, with wide media attention, teeth problem is still expanding and that is because of some fundamental issues that we all need to know and teach our children. Max's book is a great resource to cover all of these issues.

Thank you, well done.

Dr. E. Taebi, DNM, D. ACU, IET.
Spiritual Healer, Hypnotherapist

This is the first book I read that tells me why do it, what to do and how to do it to keep my teeth healthy. It is well organized and clearly written so anyone can understand it. No more excuses for not looking after your teeth. Congratulations!

Thomas Duyck, P. Eng.
Webmaster, Society of Internet Professionals, Toronto

Max Haroon has compiled a sensible, easy to read book of instructions on how to avoid the pitfalls that sabotage our natural roadway to health and wellbeing. The reader easily recognises simple mistakes most of us make and is given an easy to follow route to correct them. This book is a welcomed addition to the sign posts to that end.

Phil Fields, Health and Wellness Educator

Reading "7 Steps to Dental Health" is a gift of Self-love. These easy, natural, cost/time/life-saving recommendations show us how "dental care" opens windows into care of the whole Self. Warning: Read only if you wish to awaken more common sense and be more empowered. The practical steps outlined in the book will benefit all while self-assessment and protocols are a good resource for health practitioners.

Archana Jaiswal, MPA, Harvard. Wellness Coach and Consultant

Very impressed, with '7 Steps to Dental Health'. Max Haroon's excellent accountably and research carried throughout this book offers everyone opportunity and more understanding of holistic health. Reducing Sedation particularly resonates with me, as a Reiki Master, I've used this technique on all my procedures done on my visits to the dentist, allowing for me to avoid injection. I trust this book will bring awareness of Advance Diagnostics Tools and Trends to more and more dentists.

Rose A. Weinberg, HOM., RT-CRA, DCN, DTM, Homeopath, Reiki Master, Nutritionist, and author of "Go Forward", "the feelgood life!"

For Video Testimonials, visit http://www.youtube.com/user/7stepsdentalhealth/

Contents at a Glance

The Book Available in Different Formats
Hydroponic Sprout Grower
Sprouting Seeds and Grains to Unlock Nutrients
A Seven-Step Strategy for Your Career Success
Glossary
Index

Table of Contents

Chapter 1
A Primer on Dental Health

Chapter 2

Chapter 3
A Fresh Approach to Dental Freedom

Chapter 4
Dental Care Tools and Process

Chapter 5
Ingredients of Tooth Care Products

Chapter 6
Common Tooth Conditions and Their Remedies

Chapter 7
All About Mercury Fillings

Chapter 8
Understanding Dental Practice

Chapter 9
Assessing Your Oral Health

Chapter 10
Dentistry in the Future

Chapter 11
Food and Nutrition for Dental Health

Foreword

It is with astonishment, pride and gratitude that I have been asked to write this foreword section for what is probably the first book of its kind: a technologically advanced and yet down-to-earth holistic book on dental care.

My career at the Hippocrates Health Institute (HHI) has spanned four decades. Since those early days when I became aware of the central role that oral health plays in overall health, I have had the privilege to help thousands of people who have presented to the HHI a variety of oral health care concerns. These people have taught me that cancer, infections and even chronic fatigue syndrome can have its origins in the oral cavity.

At the HHI, we have pioneered a new approach to these all-too common conditions. First, we assess for dental toxin exposure, and then we scan for infection. Instead of adding extra dental toxins as has been the practice in allopathic dentistry (for example, mercury fillings for dental cavities), we seek out the presence of these toxins and remove them as indicated.

We have worked with people who suffered from multiple sclerosis, breast cancer and various hormone-sensitive tumours who, upon the removal of their mercury-based amalgam fillings, have reversed their disease. It pains me to know that there are an ever-increasing number of people globally suffering from these ironic missteps.

However, it is uplifting to know that there is now a comprehensive and holistic work of Max Haroon, Dr. Oksana Sawiak, Klaus Ferlow and many others on dental care. They have distilled a complex topic into a user-friendly and practical guide to better oral health. In this book, 7 STEPS TO DENTAL HEALTH, thousands of hours of front-line experience and educational research has been organized and presented in such a way as to virtually leap off the pages that follow. *7 STEPS TO DENTAL HEALTH* has become essential reading material on this extremely important subject. All of the contributors have invested their heart, souls, and minds into this literary contribution so that you can more readily understand your oral health and the deep connections that this has to the fostering of better overall health.

As Harvard University demonstrated in one of their landmark studies, the microbes in your mouth may kill you by causing cardiovascular arrest. Oral infections are so commonplace that I am sure that the overwhelming majority of you have experienced one or more in your life. Time is of the essence as in the time that it takes you to read this book, your previously placed mercury amalgams may be contributing to a host of medical illnesses. Start by opening your mouth and looking in with a mirror.

Congratulations to the authors on this most influential book on the subject of oral health.

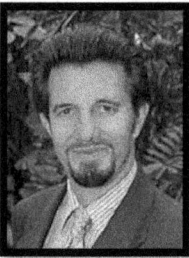

Brian Clement, Ph.D., L.N.
Hippocrates Health Institute

Brian Clement, Ph.D., L.N. Director, Hippocrates Health Institute, (USA) has spent more four decades studying nutrition and natural health care. He has received graduate degrees in both naturopathic medicine and nutritional science. Since 1980, he has directed the Institute's growth and development. Brian has conducted educational programs in more than 25 countries around the globe and is the author of numerous books including his recent best-selling book, *Living Foods for Optimum Health* **Read his profile at:** *http://www.hippocratesinst.org/*

Preface

This book is third in Life Learning Series on various aspects of life and living. This edition is a major revision and includes some new chapters while old chapters have been restructured.

The book is full of resources, which will provide additional information, other books and websites. The 1st Chapter will serve as a Primer on Dental Health, followed by the Mouth Body Connections. At the end, we will peek at the future of dentistry. The last Chapter will explore the Role of Food and nutrition for Oral and general health. A Glossary of terms is provided, which is followed by the Index.

In conjunction with its website http://7stepsdentalhealth.com, this book transforms into a multi-media resource providing extensive click-able resources mentioned in the book (so you do not have to type them). Go to Resources for Purchasers, use the user-name "book123" and password "purchaser".

Finally, appendices include additional useful information/resources to aid you in pursuing your quest for knowledge and your journey towards holistic dental health. We will start by giving you 35 Frequently Asked Questions (FAQ) with their answers. This part of the book also introduces you to the authors and contributors of the book, including the Life Transformation Institute, the publisher of the book.

This is a living book, so your comments and contributions for future editions will be highly appreciated and acknowledged. Send an email to book@7stepsdentalhealth.com and for your feedback, I will send you an advance copy of *Sprouting to Unlock Nutrients in Seeds and Grains: Grow Your Own Organic Source of Enzymes and Vitamins* as our thank you gift.

You can read this book as a passive reader and will gain some useful information, but it will not change your health. Real changes will only come if you make a conscious effort in implementing the advice given in the book.

I encourage you to share the knowledge from this book with your friends, family and dental health practitioners.

Dedication

To the special lights in my life
Sohail & Sarah

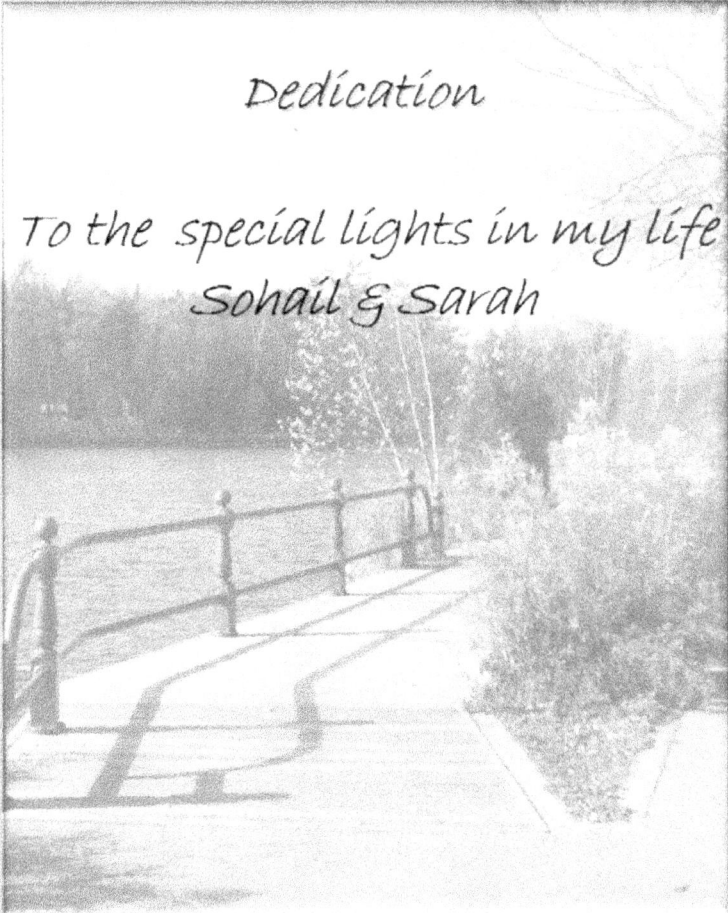

My Dental Story
Why I Wrote the Book

*'The purpose of life is not to be happy - but to **matter**, to be
productive, to be useful, and to have it make some difference that
you have lived at all".*
~Leo Rosten

My personal dental health story began about 50 years ago in England. When I heard from my dentist in his usual "You have an excellent set of teeth. There are no fillings, and there are no cavities". I was so happy! These comments allowed me to continue to eat my new-found Cadbury's chocolate bars and sugar-laden baked goods. As per my dentist's instructions, I continued brushing the way I knew (not necessarily the way it should be). I also continued to visit my dentist regularly, yet more dental work ensued, but, unfortunately, no preventive education or preventive procedures were offered.

When I left England twenty years later, about a quarter of my teeth had mercury fillings.

How had this transformation occurred? My original pristine mouth of teeth had changed to a mouth with multiple mercury amalgams. I felt disheartened and resolved to discover the cause of this change. Was there a better way to coax my gums and teeth back to their former glory? What was the connection between my diet, stress coping techniques, sleep patterns and my oral health?

Being trained as a systems analyst, I enjoyed the analysis side of problems and therefore set out to analyse my diet. I soon realized that the food I was eating was highly processed; it contained lots of refined white sugar. I had an addiction to chocolate and sodas. In light of these new revelations, simple brushing and flossing my teeth did not seem to fulfil my dental care requirements adequately.

Therefore, I changed my diet. Fortunately, I felt much better and had better oral health. Nevertheless, I was not altogether satisfied with my health or myself. I began searching for more missing pieces. I started studying stress, relaxation, and further studied the effects of food on overall health. I began to appreciate the connection between physical exercise and oral health.

After revitalizing my lifestyle and oral health, I now acknowledge that my personal dental health requires more than just brushing and flossing. The health of my teeth is affected by the health of other parts of my body; all of which are influenced not only by my choice of foods and avoidance of toxins, but also by my lifestyle and attitude in life. In this book, I venture into these interrelationships. I hope that you too can learn to see dental health as an integral part of your overall health.

I started experimenting with different brushes, rubber tips, mouthwashes and through my discovery and heuristic process I developed this seven-step system for dental care. I am happy to say that it has been a while since I sat in a chair experiencing a dental drill.

I wrote an article "Has Nature Given us the Best Tooth Design?", which led to a panel discussion in the spring of 2010. The event was a success, and led me to write this book, so others can learn from my story.

Consequently, I established the Life Transformation Institute, so I can help others on their personal journey and share my wisdom and knowledge with them. This Institute educates and shares knowledge by providing Resources, publishing Books and Hosting Panel Discussions and Presentations

I hope you will join my sojourn.

Sincerely,

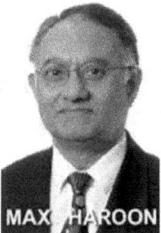

Max Haroon
Author, Founder,
Life Transformation Institute

CHAPTER 1

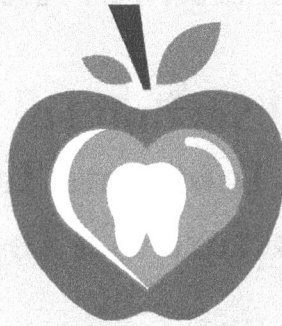

A Primer on Dental Health

You don't have to brush your teeth —
just the ones you want to keep.
~Author Unknown

This chapter will provide basics about the teeth, mouth and its relationship to systemic diseases. It will introduce holistic approach and some fundamentals to take care of your mouth.

Section 1:
Structure of a Tooth and Tooth Surfaces
Structure of a Tooth

Dentin is the solid part of a tooth, which is covered with shiny enamel on the crown (exposed part of the tooth) and cementum on the root part of the tooth. The pulp is the canal of nerves and blood vessels running inside the dentin in the tooth.

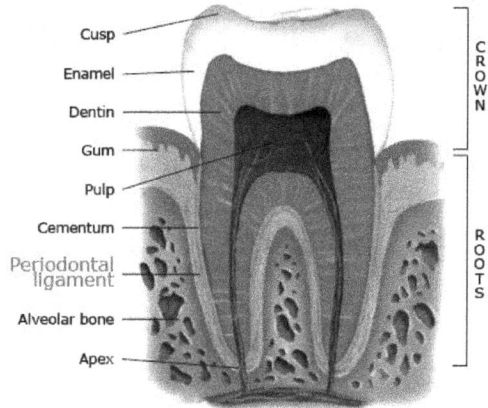

Video of Tooth Enamel

www.youtube.com/watch?v=f_Gdl0C4CnY

In addition to 32 teeth, the oral cavity also contains the following:

- Gums
- Lips
- Lining of your cheeks
- Salivary glands (glands that make saliva)
- Roof of your mouth (hard palate)

Tooth Names and Numbering

Locations of teeth and their grouping: back (molar and premolars) and front (incisors and canine).

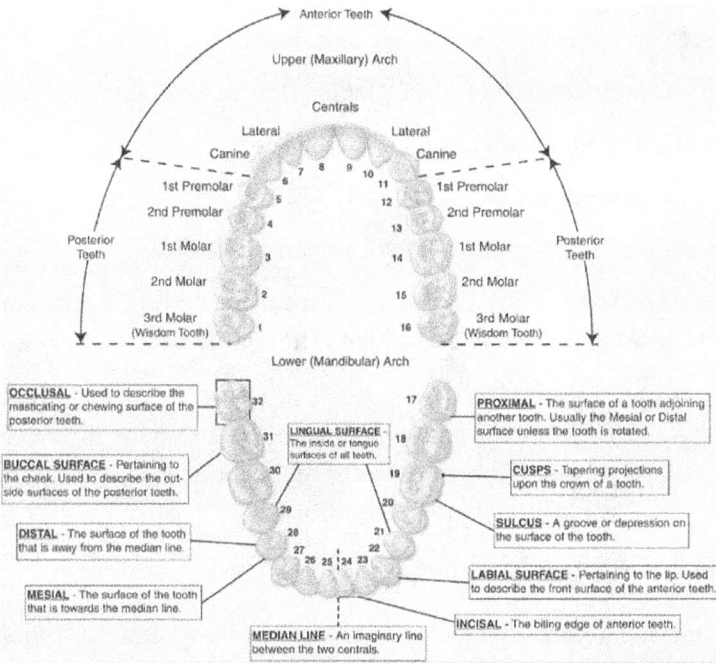

The tooth numbering system in the image above is used in the USA.

The image on the right indicates the numbering System used in Canada and UK: The mouth is divided into 4 quadrants and teeth are numbered 1-8 going from the front tooth to the wisdom tooth in each quadrant. The four quadrants are also numbered clockwise starting from upper right as 1 and teeth are numbered 1-1 to 1-8.

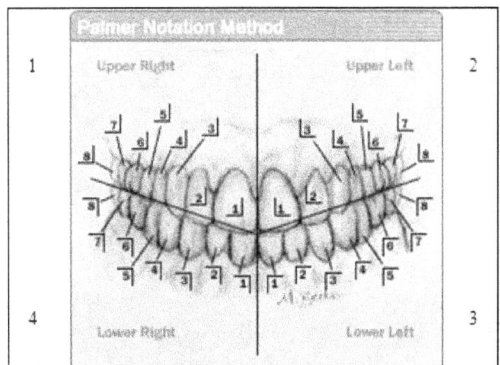

Tooth Surfaces

- There are two **arches** of teeth: upper and lower.
- Each half of the arch is called a **quadrant**, one on the left and another on the right.
- Each arch has three accessible surfaces:
  - **Outer Surface** (Buccal - facing the cheek or lip)
  - **Inner Surface** (Lingual - facing the tongue)
  - **Chewing** surface (Occlusal)
- Each arch has two "not easily" accessible surfaces:
  - The space between two teeth is called the **interdental or interproximal space** which is not easily accessible by a standard toothbrush.
  - The back surfaces of the last molar/wisdom teeth do not have any neighbouring teeth; these surfaces are only partially accessible by a standard toothbrush.

In summary, every tooth has five surfaces:

- Chewing surface (the front teeth have no chewing surface just an 'edge')
- Inner
- Outer
- Two Interdental surfaces (mesial and distal)

For the sake of simplicity, we will refer to the six anterior teeth as the 'front teeth' and all ten posterior teeth as 'back teeth' while describing brushing techniques.

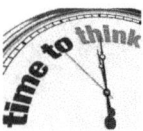

Are you thoroughly brushing and cleaning your teeth? You are if you are cleaning all the five surfaces of teeth in your mouth. Your mouth also has the following tissues and structures:

- Back of your mouth (soft palate and uvula)
- Floor of your mouth (area under the tongue)

- Tongue
- Tonsils

The Seven Steps for Oral Hygiene describe the process in Chapter 4.

Section 2:
The Story of Tooth Decay and Inflammation of Gums

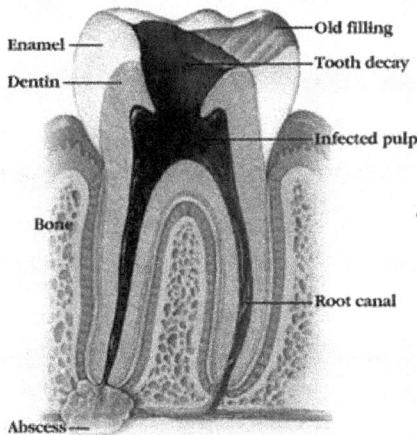

The story of tooth decay and gum disease has the following **players**:

- Susceptible Tooth (hard covering of a tooth's dentin is called enamel. Minerals are responsible for keeping the enamel hard. Pulp is the inner-most part of a tooth, see the diagram).
- Gum tissue.
- Bacteria (feed on sugar* and produce acid). There are trillions of them living in your mouth.
- Saliva (prepares food to digest and fights bacteria by keeping the acidity in the mouth low).
- Food Debris (food left over in the mouth and teeth).
- Dead Cells (from natural turnover of our cells).

- Fermentable Carbs (Carbohydrates, Sugary Food).
- Plaque (sticky acidic substance, consists of bacteria, protein and mucous).

1. When we eat, the **bacteria convert** sugary food (easily absorbable carbohydrates) into **acids**.

2. The acid dissolves the minerals of the enamel. The surface of the enamel becomes porous - tiny holes appear. After a while, the acid causes the enamel to decalcify. Once it reaches the dentine, it mushrooms into a **cavity.**

3. Live and dead bacteria, turn into a sticky substance called **plaque** that sticks to our teeth (mostly in the back **molars**).

4. If you do not brush your teeth to remove the plaque, it will **calcify** in roughly 48 hours. It will harden in almost 12 days to form **calculus or tartar.**

5. Repeated build-up of tartar will inflame the **gums.**

6. If inflamed gums are not treated over a long period, gum disease will develop called **gingivitis (first stage of a periodontal disease).**

7. Tooth decay may not show any symptoms until it is far advanced. The tooth ultimately develops sensitivity and toothache, the **pulp** (internal structure of the tooth) is destroyed, causing an abscess and finally loss of the tooth.

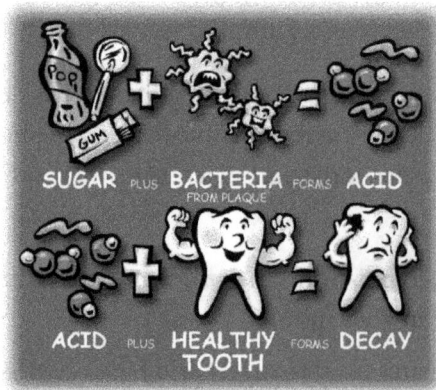

SUGAR PLUS **BACTERIA** FORMS **ACID**
FROM PLAQUE

ACID PLUS **HEALTHY** FORMS **DECAY**
TOOTH

Table sugar is not the sole source of sugar. Sugar is also found in food called simple carbohydrates (sometimes called bad carbohydrates or bad carbs), such as fruit juice, milk, honey. Details www.nlm.nih.gov/medlineplus/ency/article/002469.htm

Section 3:
A Battle Between Bacteria and Saliva

There are many causes of poor dental health, such as unhealthy food, poor lifestyle and lack of good dental hygiene. These and many other factors cause poor dental health, but who is the culprit creating tooth decay? It is the microscopic Bactria in your mouth and they are thriving in the moist warm rainforest of your mouth.

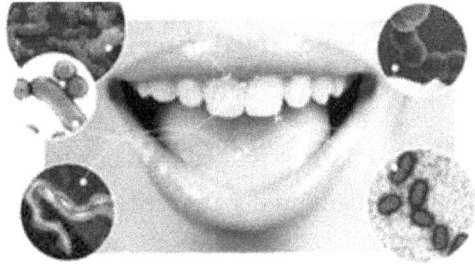

Bacteria were among the first life forms to appear on Earth, and are present in most of its habitats (animals, human and plants), soil and water. There are typically 40 million bacterial cells in a gram of soil and a million bacterial cells in a millilitre of fresh water.

In addition to your mouth, bacteria are also present in other tissues of our body, such as nose, pharynx, urethra, lower intestine, etc.

What are different types of bacteria?

They are two groups of bacteria:

- Pathogenic bacteria cause infections and
- Gut Flora or good bacteria found in the gut help to digest food.

In this section we will call pathogenic bacteria as simply bacteria. Bacteria and fungi are collectively called microbiome.

There are many types of bacteria and each part of the body have different kinds of colonies, while some are commonly present everywhere but in different proportions. Different environments/ecology and body conditions also make up different types and size of colonies.

There are two categories of bacteria in the mouth:

- Planktonic or Free floating, found in saliva
- Biofilm, found on the surface of the mouth, such as teeth and tongue

Mouth has about 60 different varieties of bacteria and they are estimated to be 10 billion bacteria in the mouth.

In this section we will talk about survival and death of the bacteria so that you can maintain decay-free teeth.

How do bacteria cause tooth decay?

When we eat, the **bacteria convert** sugary food (easily absorbable carbohydrates) into **acids** (waste product of bacteria). The acid erodes/ dissolves the minerals of the enamel. This imitates the process of decay. The surface of the enamel becomes porous - tiny holes appear. After a while, the acid causes the enamel to decalcify. Once it reaches the dentine (inner part of a tooth), it mushrooms into a **cavity.** Live and dead bacteria, turn into a sticky substance called **plaque** that sticks to our teeth (mostly in the back **molars**).

A bacterium causing most cavities in the mouth is called S. Mutans. Your mouth may contain virus if you are suffering from cold and flu or other viral conditions.

What do bacteria eat?

They survive on sugar and food rich in sugar (that includes carbohydrates). They have the availability of these foods well after you have eaten them because some food gets stuck in between the teeth, wedged between the cheek and gums and around the mouth.

Role of Saliva in Maintaining Oral Health

Saliva is a clear, slightly acidic (pH = 6.0-7.0) watery fluid which is secreted from the major salivary glands.

Saliva is the body's natural defence for the oral cavity. Saliva plays a key role in lubrication and remineralization and demineralization stages throughout the day.

Saliva contains a complex mixture of:

- Enzymes
- Hormones
- Antibodies
- Antimicrobial constituents
- Cytokines
- Buffers
- Nutritional constituents
- Mineral ions, mostly calcium and phosphate.

Testing status of these components of Saliva is a good indicator of many health conditions (such as inflammation) of mouth and body. Saliva as a diagnostic tool is described later in the book, under Advanced Diagnostics.

Since enamel of teeth also contains calcium and phosphate, the saliva helps to re-mineralize the enamel. Saliva is constantly remineralizing your teeth to fight erosion by acid. At night there is no production of saliva, so the maintenance of mouth health is compromised.

Antimicrobial factors and the buffering components of saliva can protect tooth enamel from cariogenic bacteria.

Some of the functions of Saliva in your mouth:

- Keeps your mouth moist and comfortable
- Helps you chew, taste, and swallow
- Fights germs in your mouth and prevents bad breath
- Has proteins and minerals that protect tooth enamel and prevent tooth decay and gum disease
- Helps keep dentures securely in place

Demineralization of Teeth

Demineralization (or dissolving the enamel) is the process which removes minerals like calcium and phosphate from the enamel of the tooth. Too much of demineralization can make the enamel soft, leading to a cavity.

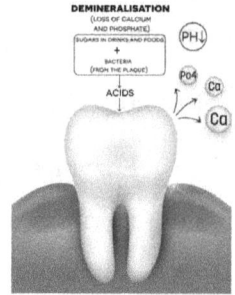

When there is acidity in your mouth, the first defence is to fight with saliva (causing dry mouth) and if that is not enough then the body pulls minerals from the enamel to buffer it.

Demineralization also occurs due to many other conditions in your mouth and body, such as stress,

How to eliminate bacteria?

You cannot eliminate them completely; no matter how intensive is your dental hygiene routine. They survive and repopulate.

Here are Seven Strategies to keep bacteria under control so that they do not damage the teeth. These and other strategies are detailed throughout this book:

1. **No Sugar:** Reduce the capacity of bacteria to produce acid by not feeding sugary/carbohydrates food and drinks.

2. **Dry Mouth:** If you have a condition or just feel your mouth is dry, then hydrate yourself by drinking water, particularly after waking up, as your mouth is dry during the sleep. You can also chew sugar-less gum made with Xylitol.

3. **Baking Soda: This is another household alkaline substance;** rinse your mouth with baking soda solution after every meal and drink.

4. **Brushing and Flossing after Every Meal:** Clean your teeth and get rid of any food debris. Follow the 7 Steps Hygiene routine, outlined in the book.

5. **Tongue Scraper;** Remove bacteria when you wake up. There is no production of saliva when you are at sleep, so the bacteria have field

night as they have no enemy to fight. You can see the evidence of that if you scrape your tongue; a thick white deposit will be on your tongue scraper.

6. **Oil Pulling:** If you wish to remove bacteria (virus too) and invigorate your gums then do the Oil pulling every morning. Take a couple of teaspoons of coconut oil (add a drop of essential oil) and swish around for 15 minutes, then spit it out. Detailed later in the book.

7. **Non**-toxic Dental Care Products: Most commercial toothpastes and mouthwashes contain ingredients such as SLS (sodium lauryl sulphate), fluoride, sodium laureth sulphate, sodium saccharin, artificial colour & scent (flavour). Instead, use non-toxic products and if unavailable then use simple household products, such as Baking Soda, salt or cranberry powder.

A whole chapter in the book is devoted to the description of these toxic ingredients and its substitutes.

I *wish you* well in your pursuit of holistic *health.*

Section 4:
Oral Health Statistics

Here are statistics on our deteriorating national health, based on some US Health Agencies; the figures are proportionally similar in Canada:

- By the age of two, nearly half the children have cavities.
- In 2004, the total mercury sold in amalgam fillings was 30.4 tons (that is 30,400 kg or 68,096 lb).
- Only 40% of the population receives dental care, and 98% need it. Unfortunately, 60% do not have the money or desire to see a dentist. The situation seems to be similar in Canada, 1/3 of Canadians do not have dental insurance according to Health Canada[1].
- By age 17, 78% of young people have had a cavity, and 7% have lost at least one permanent tooth[2].

- Among adults aged 35 to 44 years, 69% have lost at least one permanent tooth.

- Among adults aged 65 to 74, 26% have lost all their natural teeth.

- About 80% of North American adults have gum disease.

- About 20% of people over age 65 who have never smoked are toothless, while a whopping 41.3 % of daily smokers over age 65 are toothless.

- In the US, 30,000 people are diagnosed with mouth and throat cancer each year, and 8,000 die of these cancers. Although cancer screening is an integral part of an oral examination, it is sometimes missed by the hygienist or dentist.

1. ParentCentral.ca – Parenting News, Education, Family Health ... (n.d.). Retrieved from www.thestar.com/life/parent.html

2. Child Welfare League of America: Practice Areas: Health Care ... (n.d.). Retrieved from www.cwla.org/programs/health/healthtipsoral.htm

3. National Institute of Dental and Craniofacial Research (NIDCR) **www.nidcr.nih.gov/DataStatistics/**

Section 5:
Test Your
Oral-Health Knowledge

We are unaware of our poor dental health unless someone makes us aware of it or we find it the hard way from dental disease. Here are three scenarios, which can make you aware of your poor dental health.

Scenario 1: Ask yourself, "Why have you had some tooth and gum issues requiring treatment, in spite of the fact that you:

1. Brush and floss your teeth regularly

2. Eat healthy food

3. Look after yourself

4. Visit the dentist and hygienist regularly

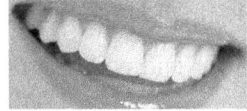

Scenario 2: Take this test to assess your dental knowledge and your dental hygiene routine.

Which one of the following is False?

1. The leading cause of tooth loss is Cavities.

2. You can thoroughly clean your teeth simply by thoroughly brushing them.

3. Eating sweets and candy causes tooth decay.

4. You can destroy tooth enamel by sucking on a lemon.

5. Chewing on ice cubes will make your teeth stronger.

6. The presence of gum disease can lead to conditions like pneumonia or diabetes.

7. You should brush your teeth immediately after eating.

Answers: #1, #2 and #5 are false.

The Explanation is available on the book's website at http://7stepsdentalhealth. com/?page_id=313

Scenario 3: Take this challenge

Do you clean your mouth 100%?

Do you access and clean every part of your personal oral structure?

I bet you think you do. If so, consider the following and you will concur with me that most people do not clean their teeth and their mouth 100%:

1. Did you brush the spaces between the teeth, by flossing or using an Interdental brush?

2. Did you remove the sticky deposits (plaque) on the gumline, particularly under the gumline?

3. Did you clean the inaccessible back surface of your wisdom tooth?

4. Did you clean back of your mouth?

5. Did you clean floor/upper palate of your mouth?

6. Did you clean your Tongue?

7. Did you use an electric brush?

Section 6:
Holistic Approach

ho·lis·tic/hō'listik/

Characterized by comprehension of the parts of something as intimately interconnected and explicable only by reference to the whole.

A holistic approach to healing recognizes that the emotional, mental, spiritual and physical elements of each person comprise a system. By working with this systems approach, the cause of an illness is targeted, rather than just the symptoms.

Holistic or Biological Dentistry is a term used for dentists who undertake a natural form of dentistry - dentistry that recognizes that dental procedures do affect the entire body.

A holistic approach to healing recognizes that the emotional, mental, spiritual and physical elements of each person comprise a system. By working with this systems approach, the cause of an illness is targeted, rather than just the symptoms.

> Amalgam Fillings: If we do not believe that the mouth is part of the body, we take a simplistic engineering approach to restorative materials – using amalgam (which is 50% mercury) for fillings, using metals such as palladium (neurologically toxic) in crowns and putting depression and allergy causing nickel crowns and braces into children and teens during their most vulnerable growing years.

Root Canal: If we do not believe that a tooth is a living organ, we embalm it with a root canal procedure and ignore the potential toxins that are released by that dead tooth over time.

Cavitations (hidden bone infections): If we do not believe that can be caused by incomplete extractions, we tell people that the pain in their jaw must be psychological or neurological. We say that the breast cancer, chronic fatigue or other condition they are suffering from have no connection to that infection deep in the jaw.

Transmission of Gum Disease: If we do not believe that gum disease is an infection that can be transmitted from person to person like a cold, then we can only treat the consequences of the infection.

Cavities and gum disease are caused by pathogens (bacteria, fungus and parasites), which are all around us. If we kiss a person who has the cold virus, and our immune system is not strong at the time, we will catch that cold. It is no different with the bacteria causing cavities or gum disease. We can catch them from another person via the use of their phone, or by being in the path of their cough, or by using a coffee cup that has not gone through a high heat dishwashing cycle after use. Even if we fly in an airplane which re-circulates the air and allows everyone's germs to be dispelled throughout the airplane, we are exposed. Many flight attendants suffer from frequent gum infections; very likely because of the exposure to germs concentrated in the re-circulated air on planes.

Implants: Implants are now the most popular way of replacing lost teeth. The concern with implants is that not only are they metal (which causes metal toxicity as discussed above) but also that there is no impervious seal between the bacteria, viruses and parasites that land in the mouth and the bone that the implant is screwed into. In my experience, most implants become infected with a low grade, silent infection, which then becomes a source of illness for many patients. In addition, neither they nor their physician, or dentist knows the cause of many conditions they develop, such as the Trigeminal Neuralgia or Burning Mouth Syndrome or ringing in the ear.

Implants using Zirconia, a biocompatible and non-metallic material, seems very promising, and has been approved by the FDA and Health Canada for over two years. However, implants are recommended only as a last resort for situations when the person has no teeth and chewing is important for eating.

Acupuncture meridians: Meridians pass through an organ, a muscle and a tooth. If a tooth has an infection, a toxic filling or crown, or has an infection left behind in the bone after an extraction, the energy of the acupuncture meridian passing through that area can be blocked. This can cause the organ or the muscle on that acupuncture meridian to develop problems. For instance, an implant on the breast meridian can cause a blockage because of the metal "screw" used in the procedure and infection can develop. Could it be a factor in that woman's breast cancer on that side of the body?

In summary a holistic dentist generally does not offer or favour the following testing and treatments:

1. Amalgam Fillings
2. Fluoride Treatment
3. Crowns
4. Sealants
5. Implants
6. Root Canal

A holistic dentist incorporates in his practice other treatment modalities such as Detox, Vitamins and Dietary supplements, homeopathy, acupuncture, ozone therapy, Infra-red devices for inflammation and pain.

A holistic dentist's approach is prevention, reduction of toxicity and using the material which are bio-compatible to the patients. They belong to associations and organisations that are proponents of such practices and follow their training and guidelines.

If we maintain a healthy life-style by practicing whole-body hygiene such as parasite elimination, total body cleanses, skin brushing, saunas, good nutrition in the form of organic, raw, enzyme-rich foods, and avoidance of sugar, empty carbohydrates, dead packaged foods

Section 7:
Seven Systems of the Body

There are many systems and functions in the human body.

Learn about them, what they do and what parts of the body are involved in that function. Learn how all systems and functions in the body are interconnected, we have shown you some interconnections with dental health in this book.

Learn how nutrients, stress, drugs and contaminants (toxic Ingredients and chemical exposure) affect various functions in the body.

Below are seven of the important systems of the body, which are readily affected by external stimulus, intakes and exposures:

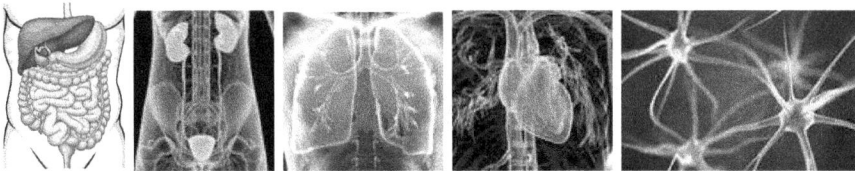

1.   The RESPIRATORY SYSTEM: To supply oxygen to the body and remove carbon dioxide. It includes the nasal passages, pharynx, trachea, bronchi, and lungs.

2.   The RENAL SYSTEM: To rid the body of waste, to regulate the amount of body fluids, and to regulate the amount of salts in the body. It includes the kidneys, the urethra, the bladder, and the ureter.

3. The CARDIOVASCULAR SYSTEM: To move nutrients, gases, and wastes to and from the body, to help stabilize body temperature, and to fight diseases and infections by transporting white blood cells to important areas. It includes the heart, blood, arteries, veins, and capillaries.

4. The REPRODUCTIVE SYSTEM: To produce eggs and sperm cells, to nurture a developing fetus, and to produce hormones. For males, it includes the testicles, seminal vesicles, prostate gland, and the penis. For females it includes the uterus, bladder, vagina, Fallopian tubes, ovaries, and the cervix.

5. The NERVOUS SYSTEM: To transmit messages from one part of the body to another. It includes the central nervous system (the brain and spinal cord) and the peripheral nervous system.

6. The IMMUNE SYSTEM: To protect the body from tumour cells, environmental substances, and invading viruses or bacteria. It includes the lymph system, bone marrow, white blood cells, and the spleen.

7. The HEPATIC SYSTEM: To break down food and store nutrients, to make proteins which are essential for blood to clot, and to purify the body of drugs, contaminants, or chemicals. It includes the liver and its veins.

Section 8:
Oral Conditions Connected to Systemic Diseases - Tooth Body Connection

Systemic means affecting the entire body, rather than a single organ, body part or a system, some such systemic disorders and diseases are diabetes and Cardio Vascular Diseases. The gum disease appears to be a local infection of the gum, however the infection can spread through the blood and can become systemic infected.

Recently, it has been recognized that oral infection, especially periodontitis, may affect the course and pathogenesis of a number of systemic diseases, such as cardiovascular disease, bacterial pneumonia, diabetes mellitus, and low birth weight. The mouth can become a port of entry for infection and site of transmission of infectious microbes. The bacteria can migrate to the lungs, digestive tract and other organs. In one recent study, people with serious gum disease were 40% more likely to have a chronic condition.

Infection and inflammation in the mouth have been linked to a variety of systemic conditions and conversely these systemic conditions can cause oral infection. We will look at the following seven systemic conditions:

1. Heart Diseases

The association of Periodontal Disease with most of the Cardio Vascular Diseases (CVD) has been well established for some time. The inflammation caused by gum disease increases plaque build-up, contributing to the swelling of the arteries. Inflammation can also cause problems in the rest of the body. It is estimated that blockages are caused by oral pathogens.

2. Diabetes

Diabetics are at higher risk for developing infections, including gum diseases. Gum disease can increase insulin resistance, thereby affecting glycemic (blood sugar) control. As per the previous section about acidity/sugar, high blood sugar provides ideal conditions for infection to grow, which can cause gum disease or aggravate it. Periodontal disease has been named as the sixth complication of diabetes.

3. Osteoporosis in Women

Bone loss in osteoporosis is also associated with gum disease and oral bone. Estrogen deficiency (in Menopause) and osteoporosis can affect the bone density, which could lead to tooth loss.

4.   Pancreatic Cancer

Researchers at the Harvard School of Public Health and Dana-Farber Cancer Institute found that gum disease *may* be associated with an increased risk of cancer of the pancreas. Research shows men with periodontal disease had a 63% higher risk of developing pancreatic cancer compared to those reporting no periodontal disease.

5.   Respiratory Conditions

Gum disease increases bacteria in the mouth. Inhaling germ-filled droplets from the mouth and throat into the lungs may cause bacterial infections. People suffering from chronic obstructive pulmonary diseases (COPD) typically lack protective systems, making it difficult to eliminate bacteria from the lungs. Patients with respiratory diseases are more at risk for pneumonia (due to the presence of cariogenic bacteria plus periodontal pathogens in their oral cavity). Elderly, who are unable to perform oral care are more at risk. Imagine how much health care cost can be saved, if all nursing home staff are trained to provide oral-care.

6.   Kidney Disease

Patients with Kidney disease are considered an "at risk" population and are more prone to infections. One of the symptoms of kidney disease is dry mouth, which is due to reduction of saliva production, which results in diminishing cleansing of bacteria, allowing bacteria to increase. This could potentially lead to the development of gingivitis and gum disease. This is a good example of systemic disease affecting dental condition.

7.   Pregnancy Condition

Studies indicate approximately 50% of women experience some degree of pregnancy gingivitis. Dental tumours, although a rare condition, are seen in the 2nd or 3rd trimester. The tumour is a painless lesion that develops in response to plaque. Pre-term delivery could be caused by periodontal gum disease and so is low-birth weight of babies born to mothers with severe gum disease.

Oral health is the most overlooked health issue in conventional and integrative medicine, but there is also some good News: It's possible to reverse cancer, digestive disorders and even diabetes by properly eliminating oral infections. Autoimmune disorders can also be resolved by getting rid of toxic dental materials.

Some diseases have oral symptoms (not necessarily caused by oral diseases) so these indicators can be used as good diagnostics tool (more on the subject in Chapter 10). The Academy of General Dentistry estimates that more than 90 percent of all systemic diseases have oral manifestations.

CHAPTER 2

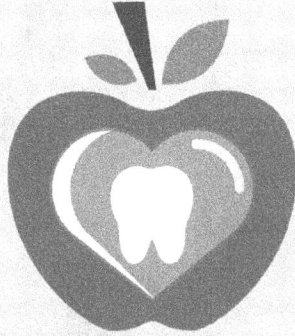

The Mouth Body Connection

Dr. Dana Colson

"Your smile radiates and reflects your inner beauty and is your best natural vitamin, a true gateway to a healthier you!"

Excerpt From: "Your Mouth: The Gateway to a Healthier You.", Dana G. Colson

In the 1950's it used to be all about the eyes, today we celebrate smiles due to the opportunity that science and research has allowed us to create beautiful smiles. Healthy smiles are paramount and when we achieve this, the byproduct is a radiant and vibrant smile.

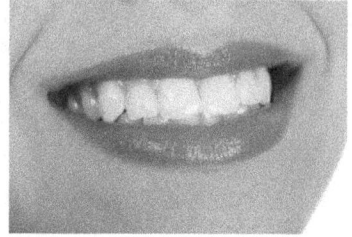

One of the ways that we communicate is through our smile. It transmits so much without any words. It is an international hello! When we smile, we give energy, warmth and honouring to others. When our muscles are activated to create our smile, endorphins are released from the limbic brain. Endorphins are our best natural vitamin. So what we give, we receive back.

Some studies show that women smile much more easily than men. One study reported that men do not smile more than 6 times a day. Surely this must change as the quality of life is important and smiling is a gift to ourselves and to others.

A prominent Canadian bank learned that 71% of Millennials would rather go to the dental office than visit a bank. Today this reflects that this generation has had positive experiences with the dentist experiencing little if any discomfort due to minimally invasive dentistry and the advantage of good home care prevention. They quest a great "white" smile as intrinsically they know the value of smiling. Advertisements and billboards show straight teeth, white smiles and happiness linked to products more than ever. The word 'smile' is often linked to banner advertisements. The integration of what dentistry can now provide is more evident than ever before. Dentistry is a major component of health that is now recognized as essential and will become a value that is a priority of wellness in future generations.

Dentistry is and will become a much more integrative approach looking at the mouth body connection. Scientists are now linking the role of inflammation with whole body health. There are direct links between periodontal disease and other serious health issues. This includes diabetes, cardiovascular disease, pregnancy complications and Alzheimer's disease. Many studies show how the bacteria in the mouth are reflected in and enhance various ailments, diseases and cancers.

A recent study showed that tooth retention helps us maintain word associations.

> Not only our mouth affects our bodily functions but also our body helps maintain a healthy mouth. We are becoming aware of how pH affects our mouth with respect to our biofilm, microbiomes, gum tissues, bone health and sustaining tooth structure.

The goal is to maintain a mouth with no gum recession, strong bone support and no more than 1 mm of wear of teeth over 100 years. As we age our teeth are vitally important for us to be able to chew our food and get the maximum nutrients from our food. The more chews we are able to do, the more enzymes are released in our saliva, allowing the digestive system to help our body and mind be strong. From a social perspective the ability to eat food and be able to converse with others at the table is important for our brain, and to share in the enjoyment of the celebration of healthy and delicious foods. To have your own soft or puréed foods due to tooth loss separates us from others and holds us back from sharing and the importance of being with our community.

Having teeth also allows us to have a proper vertical dimension for our structural physiology and allows better tongue posture to help us not be a mouth breather and reduce the possibility of snoring. Mouth breathing and often snoring lowers oxygen intake that is fundamental for our body functions, especially cardiovascular and reduces the chance of a stroke while sleeping. Nose breathing helps lower our heart and breathing rate. Our alpha brain wave activity is increased which helps us relax. Nitric oxide production is increased helping many cellular functions.

With the rapid advances of science, living to 100 may very well be the norm and 120 years of life may become the new 100. When we smile we release endorphins. Imagine having your smile as your best anti-aging part of your body. When you wake up and look at yourself in the mirror, you can say "Wow, I look great!" Seeing a wide, broad, youthful smile draws our eyes away from our wrinkles and gives us our first endorphin release of the day! Truly our smile can be our fountain of youth.

Preventative dentistry has been in the forefront of medicine for over 40 years. Good hygiene is important to sustain healthy teeth and gum tissues. Our systemic health must also be in sync. It is not enough to just brush and floss, but we need to eat healthy foods and avoid sugars and hidden sugars. Today a new form of sugar called Xylitol inhibits decay and is natural. There are many forms of sugars that take on other names and can be dangerous to our teeth even when we feel that we are making good choices. Oral bacteria create acid from both natural sugars and refined sugars. It is this acid that causes decay. An example is dehydrated fruits and power bars. They are sticky and create extensive decay even though they are thought of as "healthy snack food". Quite the contrary.

Acid reflux, GERD, the deleterious effects of some "healthy" foods, habits, swimming in chlorinated water, bulimia, tobacco chewing, and carbonated soft drinks are also destructive to tooth health. Even pure orange juice and lemon with water is very acidic and can chelate calcium and destroy our only set of "permanent" teeth. The missing piece of information that is so vital to know is that it is better to drink orange juice with calcium rather than orange juice as it does not chelate the enamel from the teeth. Lemon and water is good to drink to increase the pH levels provided you brush your teeth as soon as you awaken and prior to fluid intake. Otherwise the acid is brushed into your teeth, creating significant erosion that is not reversible. Information about what is seen in the dental world needs to percolate out to other health care professionals to enable and help others be aware of how foods and habits can destroy our teeth so that problems can be prevented at an early onset.

Many people routinely suck mints and other lozenges as they have "dry mouth" due to aging, medications or cancer treatments. It is very dangerous as they can create multiple areas of decay. When this is seen clinically, we search for the cause of the tooth breakdown and look for alternatives so this destruction does not reoccur.

Xylitol (100%) is a safe sweetener substitute as an ingredient in mints or gum to restore moisture intraoral. It not only inhibits decay, it also helps early demineralized enamel to remineralize.

Dry mouth means having no saliva or reduced amounts and an analogy is like a fish surviving without water. Saliva is vital to keep teeth hydrated and to stay healthy.

Treatment for oral cancer is surgery of the lesion, radiation and chemotherapy after the biopsy if the lesion is not in situ (fully contained). Damage to salivary glands can create dry mouth and the teeth suffer becoming more brittle and highly susceptible to decay. Early detection of cancer or dysplastic (abnormal) cells may prevent such radical treatment and extensive dental care.

Science and technology moves so quickly that the practice of dentistry is changing towards a healthy and minimally invasive mode. The digital world allows digital radiography and 3-D scanning of teeth, bone and intra-oral structures. A technology used chairside is called Velscope. It has a lens that reflects blue light and can detect cell dysplasia, or oral cancer in its early stages and also gives us information about the extent of how much the area has spread laterally.

People today are demanding more information and want to be informed about how they can integrate food for wellness and the implications on their oral health. The world has changed as our society now wants to know what is in their foods and seeks answers about what is occurring in their mouths and how to create great smiles. Labels containing ingredients and percentage of contents will become "go to" information that people will use to increase knowledge about what they consume and its effects on their mouth and body.

Just as we read the labels on foods, we will demand to know what the ingredients are in our dental materials. For example, a crown is not like all other crowns. Some are made of non-precious metals, others are high content gold and others have no metals at all. Non precious metals are less expensive and are often used in third world countries. Crowns can now be ordered from China to help offset the cost of dentistry to the consumer, however knowing the content of the product is important.

Unfortunately the material content is often not questioned. The trend is towards no metals in the mouth not only for esthetics which appeals to the public but it also lowers the electromagnetic galvanic action which occurs intraoral. To date dentistry has been using various materials which pass the test of durability, yet not necessarily what is the best for the person receiving the restoration. Today, our society has identified sensitivities as true medical concerns unlike 20 years ago when they were not in the "radar" of medicine. Mixed alloys will be used less frequently as newer materials are emerging and can equal durability intraoral. The days of highly reactive materials such as palladium and nickel mixed with gold and non-precious metals will fade out of use. With less loss of teeth, the need of various replacement appliances diminishes. The use of silver mercury restorations is already in decline. Replacement with safe protocol often eliminates the "metallic" taste. The brain fog can be reduced and energy has been seen to improve helping an individual to respond better to other therapies and be clearer for increased concentration of tasks and thought processes.

In the past gradients of health were not acknowledged as they are today. You were either allergic or there was nothing wrong with you. Over the years lactose intolerance has become the norm and gluten sensitivity has been recognized as affecting some people's health.

Our population is becoming more sensitive to materials and electromagnetic frequency disturbances. The alternative medical community has been talking about this for several decades. They quest for modalities to optimize the individual's immune response beyond the traditional tests for crisis medicine. Various remedies or lifestyle changes can increase the immune response and help a person have the ability to navigate into a better quality of life. Eastern and native modalities along with homeopathic remedies can often activate the bodily response with little if any negative side effects.

A great smile to the public means white and straight teeth.

A great smile to the dentist is firstly a healthy mouth, no decay and healthy gum tissue. A healthy foundation is fundamental to create a lasting result.

Dentists use the above criteria and then add the opportunity to create a levelled, wide and broad smile to enhance the physiology of the skeletal structure and maximize airway. Exercises of the soft tissue are helpful adjuncts that support this form of dentistry. Light gentle forces move teeth with less resistance and alignment in the mouth is reflected elsewhere in the body. Yoga exercises for the mouth and face can enhance our fountain of youth. Interestingly, Brazilians believe that having a beautiful smile means to an employer that this person will be a healthy worker.

Awareness is growing about the price we pay for grinding and clenching our teeth. We now know that yellow teeth do not have to belong to older people. We also are dispelling the myth that age creates "long in the teeth" and receding gums. People do not want to have their teeth in a glass but within their mouth for dignity during their life and on their death bed.

As wearing a seat belt for prevention while driving is now our norm.... Wearing a biteplate (also known as night guards, mouth guards, occlusal splints) for those who grind and clench will become the standard of practice even if it is episodic. It is difficult to tell when we may grind and clench at night due to our unconscious state while sleeping. However if we do grind and clench, the quality of sleep is affected dramatically and the results on teeth can be disastrous. Snoring at any age is not ideal and often is concurrent with grinding to help open up the airway for more oxygen uptake.

In the near future the population will see that a bite plate is more than protecting teeth. It helps us achieve better quality of sleep with less muscle activity in our cheeks and forehead area constantly being contracted interfering with the depth and calm of sleep. Over 70% of all headaches are tension headaches. These can be eliminated by wearing a biteplate at night and not clenching during the day. When we can keep the back teeth from touching, the temporalis muscle cannot be activated. It is when this muscle contracts that the blood flow is impeded creating head-aches. Night guards can also help increase nasal air intake dependent on design at night supplying deeper oxygenation to the body, and increasing nitric oxide intake.

Teeth should never touch. Repeating this mantra "Lips together, teeth apart and tongue in place" helps to create awareness and modify unconscious habits. When we are eating there is food between our teeth, the cusp tips of our teeth interconnect to masticate our food and then we swallow. At night the teeth are protected with a night guard. Today's society is more aware of the damage they may do when seeing intraoral pictures of their worn teeth or fracture lines within their teeth on a computer screen chairside at the dental office.

Dentists evaluate the appropriateness of a night guard making sure that one's patient neither snores nor has sleep apnea. If so, then a different diagnostic is in order and another type of mouth apparatus is called for, collaborating together with a sleep medical doctor. Again this becomes an integrative approach between professionals to help not only the mouth stay intact but help the restorative factors of the body during sleep. Many body functions including regulating blood pressure, overeating tendencies and cardiovascular health can be compromised. Sleep apnea can reduce our lifetime up to 8 years and must be treated. The gold standard is to use oral sleep appliance treatment for mild to moderate apnea.

Dentists today are being trained to look at faces to detect if there is any sign of sleep apnea, enlarged neck may have excess fat pads to obstruct the oxygen flow while sleeping, dark circles under eyes shows poor quality of sleep, and narrow dental arches with high vaults of the palate indicates low tongue posture that often shows visibly as a "double chin".

Palpating the head and neck for enlarged thyroid and lymph glands is part of what dental professionals are trained to do at each recall visit. Creating wide broad and balanced smiles can help reduce or eliminate snoring, mouth breathing, grinding and clenching and allow better physiological adaptive capability of our body. Other factors in the throat and neck may hinder resolving the snoring issue.

Truly, the mouth is connected to our body as around the 35th day in utero the mouth is formed. The fetus develops around the head and the cells intercommunicate and divide at an astonishing rate. When we are born we become linear. However the body never forgets. The mouth can detect 20 microns, the thickness of a human hair... Any variance or change intraoral can affect the human body exponentially. Professional athletes recognize this and look at every part of the body to be in harmony to maximize the best result. Hence recently there is an emphasis on the design and construction of professional mouth guards. Not only do they protect the teeth, but help maximize athletic performance guiding the lower jaw into its optimized position for best performance.

Having orthodontics when a teenager is not only a once in a lifetime activity.

Often remodeling of a smile is integral for tooth conservation if wear and tear has occurred. It can be a sign that structurally the teeth are not in the best place and thus have shown signs of excess wear and destruction.

Today we can often move teeth to their ideal position. Often teeth that were designated for restorations need less preparation or can function well with no build up necessary! A minimal tooth reduction will be necessary after movement through orthodontics to rebuild a dentition conditional on each situation, as new materials for crowns and veneers can be very thin and strong. Bonded cements enhance retention. Some materials can inhibit decay. The less tooth reduction the stronger the bond as enamel will be left rather than dentin which is more porous. This protects the pulpal tissues with less chance of teeth dying necessitating the need for either root canal treatment or extraction and then future tooth replacement.

Orthodontics does not always mean wires and brackets. Many tooth movements can be accomplished with clear aligners that are not visible to others. They do not interfere with one's personal quality of life.

Light gentle forces create the opportunity of tooth movement without a "push back" force effect. It minimizes root resorption and is painless. Today with the aid of clear aligning technology, we can often place teeth in their ideal position and if the anatomy and form need enhancement then we can add composite bonding or thin porcelain-like materials to the teeth bonded to the enamel that is incredibly strong with minimal tooth reduction. This gives us the security of strength and longevity. Matching tooth colour and texture can be achieved with the materials and techniques available today.

The better the dentistry with the use of technology aiding us to be minimally invasive means less dentistry in the future.... It will be more about co-diagnosing and co-treatment planning with modern advancements. Routine monitoring of 3-6 month re-care appointments will allow optimization so that your smile will indeed be your fountain of youth and enhancing a healthier body.

To heal others means that we must educate others to heal themselves. It is what we ourselves do on a daily basis that is important - not only what we are prescribed from our doctor until our next visit. We must become aware of how we feel, what we eat, how we move our bodies, monitor the quality of our sleep, look at where we hold tension and be able to let go or find aids to help us restore an ideal and optimal equilibrium. Meditation, yoga and awareness are tools that western society is embracing to tap into our own inner resources to honour ourselves.

The impact of our mouth on the power of words, speech and communication is both silent and spoken. I continue to be amazed at how the mouth–as the instrument for the delivery of a healthy and confident smile–can encourage our greater self–esteem and optimize quality of life.

We have more research and ability to resource answers of the mouth body connection than ever in the history of mankind.

CHAPTER 3

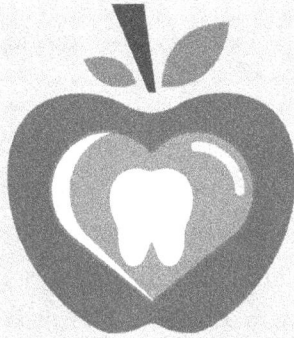

A Fresh Approach to Dental Freedom

Dr Oksana Sawiak

The man with a toothache thinks everyone happy
whose teeth are sound.
~*George Bernard Shaw*

Section 1:
Introduction

Staying healthy is a full-time job! Regaining health is a gargantuan one - sometimes too daunting for people to undertake, so they choose the "quick fix" symptom-relief path that conventional medicine offers. So starts the downward spiral of drug side effects, management of chronic illness and general decline in quality of life until we end up in the nursing home, unable to enjoy the full life we were meant to have until at least the age of 100.

Dr. Weston Price was a prominent dentist and founder of the Research Institute of the National Dental Association. His research proved that infections from teeth and gums cause a myriad of illnesses. So many illnesses, from arthritis to heart disease, from miscarriages to brain abscesses can be linked to poor dental hygiene. Dr. Price showed with his study of primitive societies that robust dental and physical health goes hand in hand with nutrition and life choices. The most harmful factor he found was refined food in the form of white sugar and white flour which caused decay, abscessed teeth and gum infections. These in turn affected the health of the whole body. Many researchers, including Dr. Rosenow of the Mayo Clinic and, more recently Dr. Boyd Haley of the University of Kentucky validated his results.

During my own 42 years of dentistry, I strove to make a difference in the health of the person behind the teeth. Much of the time, I had to convince my patients that not only were their teeth crucial to their general well-being, but also if their teeth got sick, the entire body got sick. After retiring from active dentistry, I still continue to teach the safest way to health through Wellness Consulting. Though many dentists still believe that they can do ANYTHING to the patient's tooth - like root canals, toxic crowns and fillings, and implants - with impunity; more and more are embracing the truth that teeth are indeed a part of the body, and a hugely important one at that.

Holistic Dentistry is a term used for dentists who undertake a more natural form of dentistry - dentistry that recognizes that dental procedures do affect the entire body. But if you seriously think about it, *every dentist is holistic* since they do affect the entire body with

the materials they use and the procedures they employ whether they realize it or not; whether they admit it or not. The Standard Dentist just does not realize the extent of that effect because his/her beliefs are based on what was taught in dental school and what is still continued to be taught under the concept of Standards of Care. I prefer the term Biologic Dentist for the professional that bases his/her procedures on science and on the Hippocratic Oath – "At least do no harm".

The reason **Biologic Dentistry** is not the standard of care is that dental schools do not stress the *health* aspect of the profession. They tend to follow the fragmented allopathic medical model that each part of the body functions separately as if in a vacuum and treatment is all about relieving the symptoms. Therefore, the stress is on root canals for painful teeth, fillings for cavities, crowns for broken teeth, and cutting away gums that are sick rather than curing the infection. *Healing, supporting* and *preventing* are biologic concepts. Getting "the carpentry on the tooth" exact - right down to one tenth of a millimetre - is the standard allopathic approach.

Similar to the biologic dentists, there are also biologic hygienists or holistic dental hygienists; in fact, they spend more time in preventive education than dentists do at schools.

Do not blame your dentist for following the standard, allopathic, accepted model since he/she is merely trying to keep their dental license, keep the peace with the profession and feed his/her family. Now it is up to the consumers, we the patients, to demand the change.

The way that the standards in dentistry will be changed in the future is by the demands which the general population makes of dentists, insurance companies and the regulatory bodies. Already we are seeing a huge reduction in the placement of mercury amalgam fillings because most people demand "white" fillings rather than "silver" ones. Many people are surprised when they find out that mercury amalgams are still in use at all. Because some European countries have banned them, North Americans think Canada and the US have banned them as well. Not only has this not happened, but also since 1996, Health Canada's Position Statement on Dental Amalgam, which advises dentists to avoid placing amalgams in children and women of childbearing age, has not been honoured by most dental offices. Most dental personnel do not even know what the position of Health Canada is on dental amalgams.

Unfortunately, the poor and disabled who have to rely on Public Health Services do not get a choice. They get mercury amalgams placed in their teeth when fillings are required.

Section 2:
What Is Wrong With The Conventional Approach?

If we maintain a healthy life-style by practicing whole-body hygiene such as parasite elimination, total body cleanses, skin brushing, saunas, good nutrition in the form of organic, raw, enzyme-rich foods, and avoidance of sugar, empty carbohydrates, dead packaged foods and toxic GMO products, we will be much more resistant to the germs around us. The soil and conditions for germs will be infertile and unwelcoming. There will be no deep, dark putrefying areas to land and grow in.

Candida is a particularly common factor in what Dr. Graeme Munro-Hall calls MAD – Modern Chronic Disease. Candida is a fungus that is opportunistic, meaning it flourishes when conditions are right for it to grow and prosper. It grows where the normal flora (good bacteria) have been disturbed, for instance by antibiotics or toxins (e.g. Mercury) or high-sugar diets. Candida causes gum recession and rapid decay at the gum line if not eliminated or controlled.

When we accept a prescription from a physician for an antibiotic to deal with a non-life-threatening condition like a cold, and we do not restore the balance of our gut flora with probiotics, we set ourselves up for many other uninvited complications. Many cancer patients do not die from the cancer itself; it is the Candida infection that kills them.

So what can we do to help ourselves? This book is an excellent base starting point.

Oral hygiene of course is utterly necessary and Max Haroon has well outlined all the details, in chapter 4, of accessing and cleaning every part of our personal dental structure. He has emphasized the life-style choices people need to make to restore and maintain dental health as well as to prevent the world's most common diseases: cavities and gum disease.

CHAPTER 4

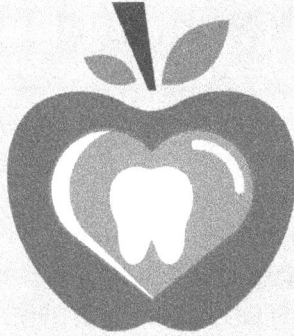

Dental Care Tools and Process

Dentist: a prestidigitator who, putting metal into your mouth,
pulls coin out of your pocket.
~Ambrose Bierce

Section 1:
Has Nature Given us the Best Tooth Design?

When it comes to teeth, nature has not given us the Best Design!

I do not think it is an easy task to clean and maintain healthy teeth, considering the shape, accessibility of teeth or their surfaces, the junction between teeth and gums, and spaces between the teeth.

You would think brushing or flossing should do the job!

What about the sticky deposits? What about cleaning the junction between the teeth and gums?

> The dirtiest place in the body we would think would be the colon or bowels, but actually, it is the mouth, especially the tongue which is literally teeming with pathogenic micro-organisms.

Even if we use a toothbrush to remove these bacteria, many still remain and repopulate the mouth.

Brushing your teeth with a popular brand toothpaste still leaves 40-70% of the pathogenic microorganisms hidden around your teeth and on the tongue.

There are a few key factors involved in cleaning the teeth:

- Removing food particles from all tooth surfaces, in between the teeth and off the tongue.

- Removing plaque or 'the sticky film' from your teeth: Imagine magnetic iron powder attached to a metal tooth. Do you think you can brush all the iron powder from the metal tooth? No, you have to "demagnetise" it or shake the iron powder off. Plaque is similar to that sticky iron powder (it has an electrical positive charge).

- Killing harmful bacteria.

I have designed my own process to clean my teeth and mouth based on my heuristic approach, a lifelong learning process of trial and error.

This seven-step process focuses on the process and not on techniques. It includes the various stages of brushing with different types of toothbrushes and "scaling" with different devices. The process ends with some simple touches which have a therapeutic effect upon your oral health.

If you follow the process, after every meal or at least twice a day, then you will reduce the number of much-dreaded visit to the dentist or hygienist. Your options are to protect your teeth from decay and your gums from infection or to face a close encounter with the dentist's drill or a hygienist's scaler.

A word of caution, do not expect healthy teeth and gums if you are already suffering from any tooth decay and gum disease. First, get your teeth and gums treated and then follow this regimen for maintaining your oral health.

We will begin with a short description of tooth care products, followed by my Seven Steps for Oral Hygiene.

Section 2:
Dental Hygiene Tools

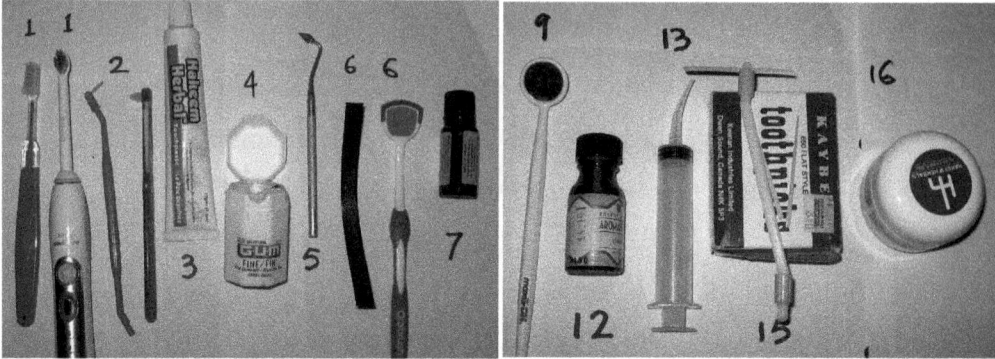

Your dental hygiene kit should include the following tools:

1.　Toothbrushes (Manual and Electric)

2.　Interdental Brush

3.　Toothpaste

4.　Dental Floss

5.　Rubber Tip Stimulator

6.　Tongue Scraper

7.　Essential Oils

8.　Baking Soda

9.　Dental Mirror

10.　Disclosing Tablets

11.　Hydrogen Peroxide 3% (mainly for sterilizing)

12.　Mouthwash

13.　Oral Irrigation Syringe

14.　Salt

15.　Toothpicks (use sparingly with approval of your dentist) and softpicks

16.　Tooth Powder

These tools are discussed briefly here and also in the next section.

1. Toothbrushes

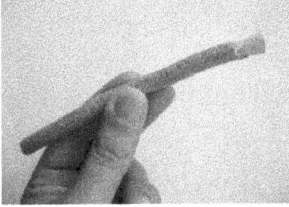

In traditional cultures, such as Indian and African, people chewed on soft twigs of trees such as neem or peelu, making the tip of the twig like a brush to clean their teeth and massage their gums. These improvised brushes known as siwak or miswak, were highly effective. Those people kept their teeth healthy for life.

It is preferable to use a small headed toothbrush with "soft" rounded nylon bristles so you can reach the small areas where those nasty germs like to hide. A brush head with three rows of bristles is wide enough for an adult (see the image). Most brushes need to be replaced after three months use (when they are splayed or infected).

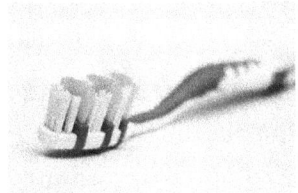

There are many types of manual toothbrushes:

- Standard toothbrush.
- Three-row brush (you will find them in the children's section, they are recommended for adults).
- Two-row sulcus toothbrush (to reach between the gums and the teeth).
- Special action toothbrush (such as Ionic or Blotter).
- Interdental brushes (also called proxy, proxa or interproximal brush); they are designed to clean in-between the teeth. Use of the Interdental brush is explained in Step 3 of the Section 5: Seven-Steps of Oral Hygiene.

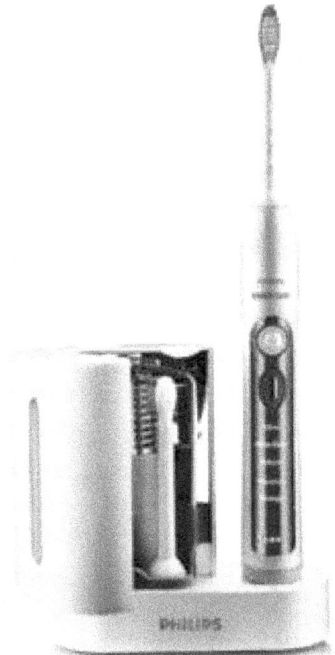

- Electric toothbrush; according to some research, electric toothbrushes remove 50% more plaque in comparison to manual brushes. You can adjust the pressure and vibrations with many of the electric brushes.

Your kit should include a variety of brushes and an electric brush.

Most of the manual brushes are available as soft, medium and hard bristles but soft brushes are usually recommended.

2. Interdental Brush

Interdental brushes are also referred to as proxy brushes, proxa brushes or interproximal brushes. They are designed to clean in-between the teeth, they come in various sizes and shapes. Some of them are disposable and some with refills to change the brush head.

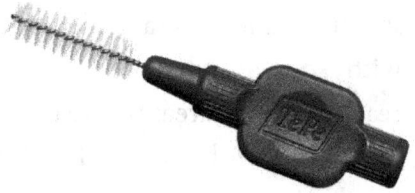

The use of an Interdental brush is only advisable for people who have enough space in between teeth (which can happen if you have had surgery or recession due to some gum disease or a gap due to extraction of a tooth).

3. Toothpaste

Like mouthwash, it is better to use a toothpaste with natural ingredients. Avoid one with toxic substances like sodium lauryl sulphate (SLS) and propylene glycol. Avoid fluoride toothpaste as well (controversial with standard dentistry). Chapter 5 outlines various toxic ingredients in commercial toothpastes.

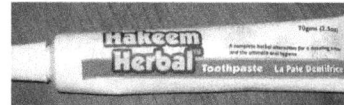

Instead of toothpaste, you sometimes may use essential oils or a baking soda solution. Section 7 of this chapter describes recipes for natural toothpastes and mouthwashes.

4. Dental Floss

Dental floss is a thread (cotton or nylon) used to remove food and dental plaque from teeth. It can be waxed or unwaxed in a dispenser or on a handle.

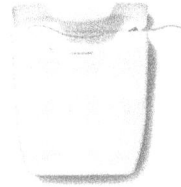

5. Rubber Tip

Despite all the claims by toothbrush vendors (manual or electric), you cannot remove all the plaque from your teeth with a toothbrush.

A rubber tip can be used at or below the gum line without damaging the gums. Use of the rubber tip is one of the seven steps in our Seven Steps of Oral Hygiene (Section 5). If you clean regularly with the rubber tip at least twice a day, you will prevent build-up of plaque.

Hygienists are experienced and trained to use various types of metal scalers. Do not use a metal scaler yourself. Instead use a rubber tip. Some toothbrushes have a rubber tip built into the handle or you can get a rubber stimulator with removable rubber tips.

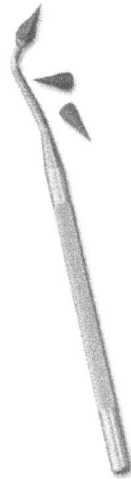

6. Tongue Scraper

It is used to clean off the bacterial build-up, food debris, fungi and dead cells from the surface of the tongue. Bad breath is often caused by bacteria at the back of the tongue where the bacteria and bacterial plaque produces sulphur odour.

There are many types of tongue cleaners. They come in different shapes. Even a small stainless steel teaspoon can be used as a tongue scraper.

7. Essential Oils

Essential oils are the pure essence of the plants and can provide both psychological and physical benefits when used properly.

Your oral hygiene could be vastly improved simply by adding proven and potent antiseptics that are safe and natural and kill bacteria, fungus and parasites.

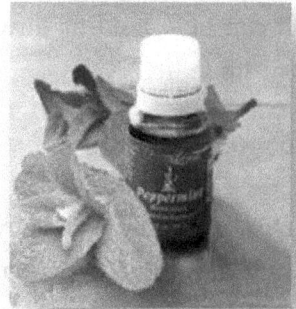

Essential oils with antiseptic and antibacterial properties that are often used for oral hygiene include peppermint, wintergreen, eucalyptus, thyme, clove, lemon, cinnamon, oregano and rosemary.

The Journal of the American Dental Association has documented over 100 studies on the effectiveness on how essential oils kill microbes that cause tooth decay and gingivitis.

Essential oils of thyme, clove, and cinnamon possess significant inhibitory effects against 23 different types of bacteria.

In fact, **thyme** oil is one of the strongest antiseptics known. Researchers found that thyme kills over 60 different strains of bacteria and 16 strains of fungi. A small amount of thyme oil will kill pathogenic organisms for tooth decay, gingivitis and bad breath.

Essential oils have proven to be even more effective than FDA recognized plaque-control drugs, such as fluoride. A 1999 study published in the Journal of Clinical Periodontology found that an essential oil mouth rinse containing thymol, menthol and eucalyptus was far more effective than an antiseptic mouthwash with fluoride.

Even mainstream dentistry for decades has used essential oil **of clove** for its antiseptic, analgesic and anti-inflammatory properties to numb gums and kill infection.

Another study revealed that individuals who used an essential oil based mouthwash twice daily had 34% less plaque build-up and better oral hygiene compared with a control group. The essential oils used were thyme, peppermint, wintergreen and eucalyptus.

A Word about Oil of Oregano

One of the most powerful and effective oils for toothache is oil of oregano. The most active ingredient in wild oregano oil is Carvacrol, a potent, naturally occurring compound that has remarkable effects against all types of microbes such as bacteria, virus, fungus, and parasites. Carvacrol can range from as low as 20% as the active ingredient in oil of oregano to a natural high of 87%; Orega Hemp has 86%. The percentage of Carvacrol content can make a significant difference in the overall effectiveness of oil of oregano. Recent studies have shown positive results and attest to the effective use of Oil of Oregano for medicinal purposes over the centuries. The oil benefits Athlete's Foot, insect bites, rashes, burns and lesions, cold sores, acne, eczema, nail fungus, warts, arthritic pain, dandruff, psoriasis, sore throats, bronchitis, sinus, chest congestion, ear and mouth infections, Candida, travel bugs, and salmonella (food poisoning). Oil of oregano also boosts the immune system.

A brand called Orega Hemp is oregano oil infused in certified organic hemp oil because oil of oregano is too strong by itself.

8. Baking Soda (Sodium Bicarbonate)

Baking soda is the rising agent in baking powder and has a history in cleaning teeth; it was used in tooth powders around the 18th century.

Towards the end of the 19th century, tooth powders using baking soda were mass-produced. Baking Soda is alkaline (refer to Chapter 11 for discussion of alkalinity and acidity). It neutralizes the acidity of the mouth and kills bacteria. You can use it as mouthwash (mixed with water) or apply with your finger/brush to clean your teeth.

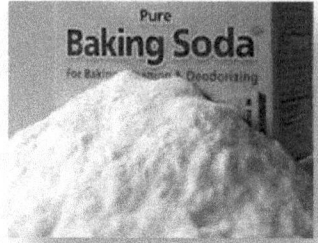

9. Dental Mirror

Dental mirror allows you to see the inside of your mouth and most of the tooth surfaces in a well-lit bathroom mirror. Examine for any bleeding, swelling, plaque and stain build-up. A dental mirror is also useful, particularly after using a disclosing tablet.

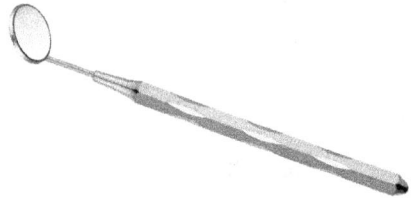

10. Disclosing Tablets

They are valuable to examine the areas of the teeth where you are missing brushing or where there is a build-up of plaque. These tablets stain plaque so that where you have missed will show up as red or dark. You can use a rubber tip or a toothpick (in a handle) to clean these areas.

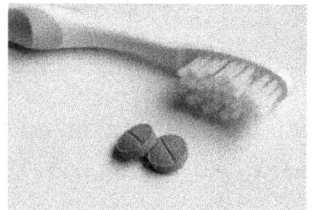

11. Hydrogen Peroxide

Hydrogen peroxide (H_2O_2) is available from 3% (most commonly available) to 35% (food grade). It kills bacteria, viruses and fungi on surfaces and is a handy and inexpensive chemical for sterilizing brushes and other dental tools. It has been used effectively as a mouthwash but it is not advisable if you have amalgam fillings or metal in your mouth. Please note that 35% peroxide can cause severe burns and must be handled carefully.

For more information

www.actualcures.com/hydrogen-peroxide-prevents-new-cavities-ends-gingivitis.html

12. Mouthwash

Avoid any mouthwash with alcohol and toxic chemicals. You can use salt water or make your own with baking soda and salt (some simple recipes are given in Section 7).

Chapter 5 outlines various toxic ingredients found in commercial dental products.

13. Oral Irrigation Syringe

It is a handy tool to access an infected periodontal (gum) pocket or a hole in your gum after an extraction. A syringe can also be useful to deliver a variety of healing solutions that can be helpful in treating gum disease or just to flush out the pocket.

14. Salt (Sodium Chloride)

Salt (NaCI) is the most common and abundant material in the world found in rocks, sea and salt lakes. It is predominately sodium chloride (our body cannot produce sodium and chloride); it also has other trace minerals (sulphate, magnesium, calcium, potassium, bicarbonate, bromide, borate, strontium, fluoride). Both table and sea salts may require significant processing to remove impurities. Sea salts retain the trace elements while table salt has been processed to remove trace elements and contain additives and iodine. Many microorganisms cannot live in an overly salty environment. Salt is used in toothpaste, mouthwashes, and rinsing dental hygiene tools due to its cleansing and disinfectant properties.

15. Toothpick or Soft Pick

A toothpick is a small, thin stick of wood or plastic which is used to remove plaque or food debris from the tooth with its pointed end. You cannot access nooks and crannies with a toothbrush, but you can with a toothpick or a soft pick (thin brush with a minute handle). It is difficult to reach back molars or inner surface of your teeth without using a toothpick handle (such as Perio-Aid) to hold the toothpick. Use the toothpick sparingly with approval of your dentist

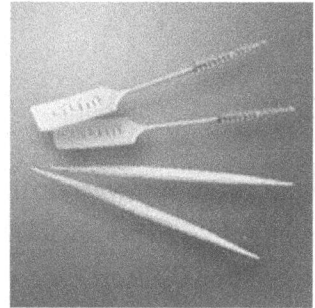

A toothpick is handy when you want to clean food debris immediately after a meal when eating out, but the use of a toothpick is not a substitute for brushing or flossing.

16. Tooth Powder

The dry dental powders are not often used these days but historically they were used before the advent of toothpaste. They are still available for uses such as whitening and gum treatment. You can make your own tooth powder as described in Section 7 of this chapter.

Basic Dental Hygiene Kit

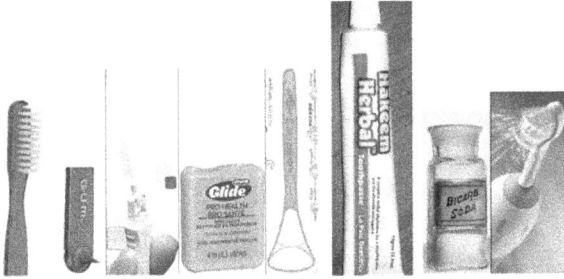

You need the following basic tools to perform the correct oral hygiene:

1 Toothbrush

2 Rubber Tip

3 Interdental Toothbrush (Sliding hinge system allows you to change the angle)

4 Natural Toothpaste (free from Fluoride, SLS, other toxicity)

5 Dental Floss

6 Tongue Scraper

7 Baking Soda

8. Electric Toothbrush

We have assembled a small kit for you, packaged with the book. Visit the book's website under "Oral Care Kit" 7stepsdentalhealth.com/?page_id=627

Section 3:
Brushing Techniques

Understanding Effective Brushing Motions

If you were to clean a comb by using a toothbrush what brush motions would clean the comb?

There are four possible, brushing motions:

1.   Going up and down along the teeth of the comb

2.   Going top to bottom only

3.   Going back and forth (sideways)

4.   Circular motion

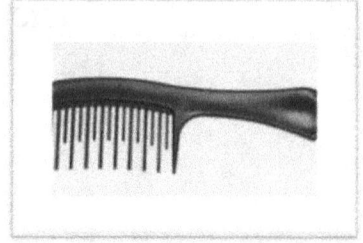

You will discover the most effective is motion # 2 (starting from the top and going to the bottom). If you go back and forth with the brush, you may be lodging the dirt back in the base of the comb. You will get better results if you angle the brush at 45 degrees, when you start from the top, and jiggle to dislodge the particles.

If there are any fine particles still stuck in your teeth you will need to use a thin pointed rubber tip or a toothpick.

We will use the same principles in brushing your teeth. First a toothbrush then a rubber tip.

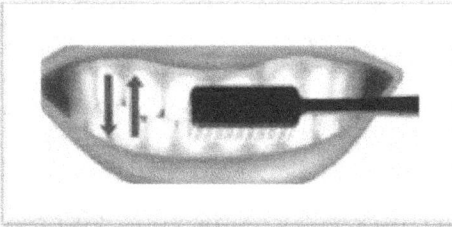

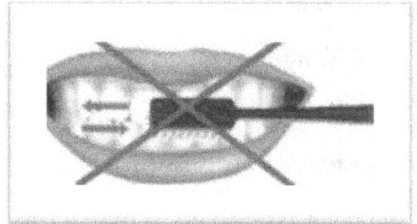

People tend to use the toothbrush by going up and down or back and forth which is not correct.

What you need to do is to align your brush, so the bristles are at a 45 degree angle at the gumline (the area where your tooth and gum meet). Jiggle your brush gently as if you are vibrating the brush covering one or two teeth at a time as you bring the brush towards the chewing surface. Starting at the gumline at 45 degrees, you are also attempting to push some bristles of the brush inside the pocket of the gumline to dislodge any plaque or food debris trapped there.

Pay more attention on inside of your lower teeth, where the plaque is found most often.

Brushing Different Tooth Surfaces

The following diagrams illustrate the angle and position of the brush for the lower arch and then for the upper arch, starting with an inner surface then outer surface:

1. **Chewing Surface: Upper & Lower Arch**

    The brush is lying straight on its bristles and your motion is back and forth. You can also brush side to side to clean small crevices (see the image).

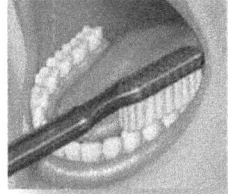

2. **Lower Arch**

    2A: Inner surface, back teeth: The brush is at about a 45 degrees angle and is making contact with the bottom of the teeth at the gumline. The motion is a slight wiggle and upwards to the chewing surface. Make sure you brush all the teeth, a couple at a time (see the image).

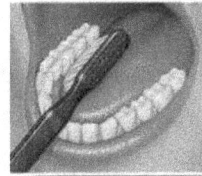

    2B: Inner surface, front teeth: The inner surface is not easily accessible, so you have to pay extra attention when brushing there. The curve in this area makes it difficult to place the width of the brush head. Therefore, hold the brush pointing straight in and down. Use the bottom of the brush head to brush the inside centre teeth. It is making contact with the bottom of the teeth and the gumline. The motion is going up towards the chewing surface (see the image).

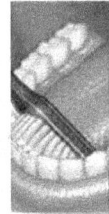

    A preferable and easier method for this area would be to use a small round, pointed-head brush, keeping the same

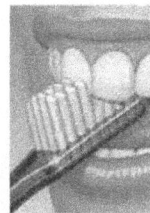

movement starting from the gumline and going towards the top of the teeth, one tooth at a time.

2C: Outer surface, back teeth: Repeat as in 2A.

2D: Outer surface, front teeth: Repeat as in 2B.

3. **Upper Arch**

3A: Inner surface, back teeth: Brush as in Step 2A. Brush is pointing downwards.

3B: Inner surface, front teeth: Brush as in Step 2B. Brush pointing downwards (see the image).

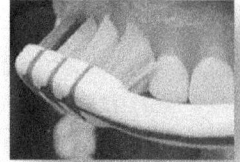

3C: Outside surface, back teeth: Brush as in Step 2C. Brush pointing downwards (see the image).

3D: Outside surface, front teeth: Brush as in Step 2D. Brush pointing downwards (see the image).

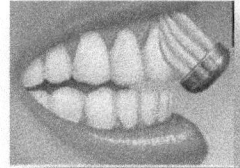

Please note

1. Divorce your mind from the association of the words "scrub" and "brush". Put a hammer in someone's hand, they want to hit something. Put a brush in someone's hand, they want to scrub something. Get over it! DO NOT SCRUB with a toothbrush.

2. Brushing is a meticulous task, *not* an athletic endeavour. For most people, it is just the opposite.

3. The object is to POSITION the bristles where you want them and then to vibrate or wiggle the brush head so that the tips of the bristles work into tiny spaces and the shafts of the bristles wipe the teeth but the brush head DOES NOT TRAVEL ANYWHERE. (This is how sonic toothbrushes work.)

It is true that some folks will gather stain on the outer surfaces (mainly due to wine, tea, coffee, tobacco, etc.) but stain does not cause disease. Such unsightly stains are easily removed with a fingertip dipped in fine baking soda.

If you want more information, there are many videos on youtube.com and videojug.com. Search for "Right Way to Brush Teeth", e.g.

www.youtube.com/watch?v=MUQevxovDSs

www.videojug.com/film/how-to-brush-your-teeth

Visit this book's website to link to some of the selected videos.

Section 4:
Seven Steps of Oral Hygiene

Purpose

The purpose of following this seven-step oral hygiene process is:

- To get rid of food debris from the mouth (teeth, tongue and cheeks)
- To get rid of plaque
- To kill harmful pathogens: bacteria, viruses, fungi and parasites
- To massage the gums

Acidic Food and Your Teeth

Most food, such as fruit, fruit juices, honey, raisins, yogurt, citrus and soft drinks and wine are acidic (low pH value), and as such they weaken the enamel of teeth.

1. Consume or drink acidic food within five minutes instead of sipping and sucking them slowly (such as sucking a lemon piece).

2. Eat them before a meal.

3. Continuous consumption of acidic food can lead to irreversible dental erosion. This is not to discourage you from eating fruits and vegetables but to learn when to eat and how to reduce their negative impact.

Read more about the Glycemic Index and pH of foods and in Chapter 11, Section 5.

In order to reduce acidity in the mouth, follow the following tips:

1. Rinse, preferably with a solution of baking soda. If you are unable to brush or rinse then just wash down your food debris after eating, by drinking a little water. The model is "swish and swallow" or "Swish and spit", depending on the setting of where you are at.

2. Eat a small piece of hard cheese.

3. Chew on sugar-free chewing gum with Xylitol, which stimulates the saliva production and reduces the acidity of the mouth as well as kills pathogens.

Step 1: Rinsing

All you need for this is a solution of baking soda in water or a natural mouthwash.

Purpose

- To clean your mouth of food debris.
- To reduce acidity, which is caused by the bacteria feasting on fermentable carbohydrates.

Tasks

1. Wash your hands with soap.
2. Rinse your teeth and swish for 15 to 30 seconds with water or mouthwash.
3. Spit out.
4. Rinse again, gargle and spit out.

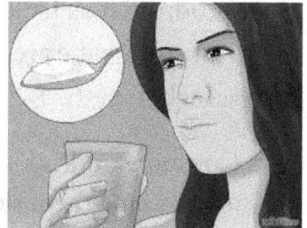

Step 2: Brushing

This is a significant step in the process, where the majority of tooth cleaning takes place.

You will need a soft-bristled toothbrush, toothpaste or tooth powder and water. Brush for two to four minutes.

Purpose

It is to remove most of the food debris and plaque.

Tasks

1. Apply just a tiny amount of toothpaste (pea size, especially if your toothpaste has fluoride).

2. Apply toothpaste evenly on your teeth (you are not brushing): Go over your teeth with a light gliding motion (no pressure or back and forth or up and down motion), starting in the centre, first the outer surfaces and then the inner surfaces of the teeth. Finally, the chewing surfaces.

3. Brush your teeth using the method explained above in section 4, one surface at a time.

4. Make sure that you brush all the surfaces.

5. Rinse.

6. Wash your toothbrush in hot/warm water.

Step 3: Interdental Hygiene

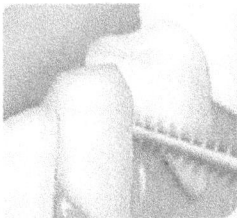

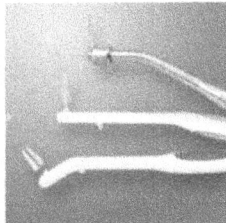

Jsing an Interdental Brush   Interdental Brushes   Soft-Picks and Tooth-picks

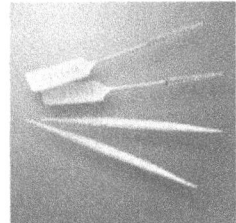

Interproximal or interdental is the name for the space between adjacent teeth. No matter how good your toothbrush is or how effective your technique, it is challenging to clean the surfaces between the teeth.

In order to clean between the teeth, you can use one of the following methods (rotate their use):

- Dental floss (preferable)
- Interdental brushes
- Toothpicks and soft picks

In this step, we will focus on flossing, which is more effective than other methods. Once a week, do consider other methods; in this way you will benefit from the rotating of different methods. Some dentists think flossing is more important than brushing and some hygienists endorse flossing prior to brushing. A suggestion is to floss after eating fruits like oranges and rinse with salted water if you do not have time to brush.

Purpose

The brushing (Step 2) may only achieve 60% of the cleaning; whereas flossing and/or Interdental brushing will do the rest of the cleaning. More than one-third of your tooth surfaces are not accessible by a toothbrush. In addition, if you get a cavity in the interproximal surface, it can only be repaired by drilling through the biting surface to get at it. Thus, even if the cavity is only attacking one surface, the subsequent filling will involve two surfaces.

Flossing

1. Pull about (30 cm) of floss from the floss dispenser.
2. Wind both ends of the floss around the middle fingers.
3. Use the index fingers and thumbs to guide and operate the floss. Leave about an inch of floss between the hands to floss between the teeth (see the image below).
4. Starting from one end of an arch, push the floss between two teeth, by gently sawing through the contact (where two teeth are touching) and move along the contour of each tooth going up and down until you hear a squeak (see the image below).

5. Gently move the floss under the gumline (see the image below) going towards the chewing surface. Do not use a shoe-shine motion. Go upwards if you are on the lower teeth (or downwards if you are on the upper teeth).

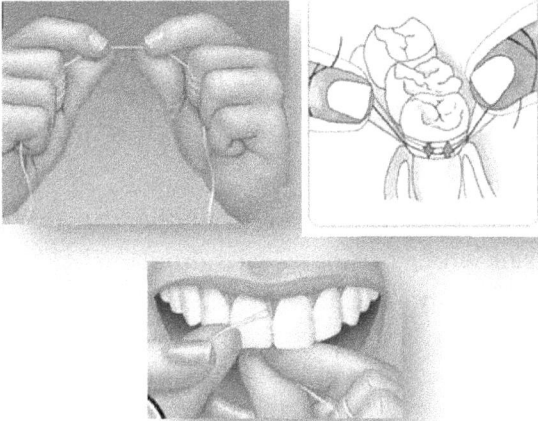

Tips

Gently glide the floss using the sawing motion to the contact point (tightest point, where two teeth touch) to reach below the gumline but make sure you do not damage or cut your gum tissues by allowing the floss to snap through the contact.

Watch videos about flossing

www.youtube.com/watch?NR=1&v=WUu-IQl5qow

www.youtube.com/watch?v=5iZfxyX6-nA&feature=related

Alternatives to Manual Flossing

There may be many reasons why more than ¾ of people do not floss their teeth. One of the reasons is the difficulty of flossing. If you are not dextrous enough to wrap the dental floss around your fingers and floss your teeth, then look into alternative methods of flossing.

- Soft-picks.
- Floss-pick (disposable): It has pre-threaded floss with a saw like handle.
- Electrical water floss (uses water jet instead of floss), also called water pick or water jet oral irrigator.

Flexible rubber bristles slide between teeth to help safely remove plaque and food particles

- Air Floss: The advantage here is that rather than having to bend over the sink letting oceans of water drool out of your mouth, the Air Floss uses only a teaspoon of water.

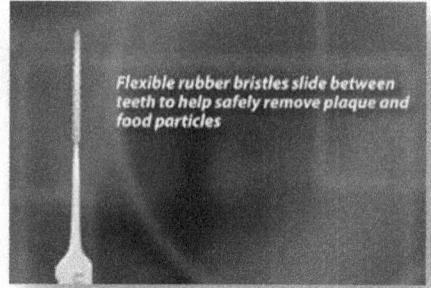

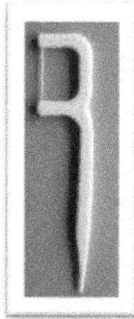

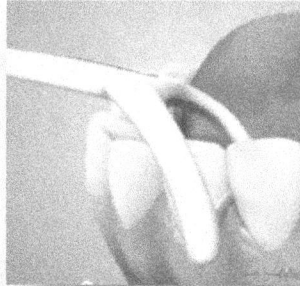

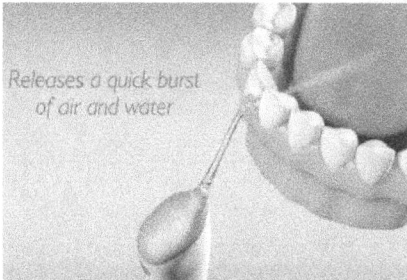

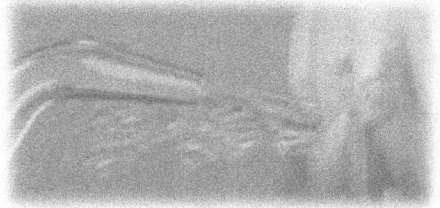

Releases a quick burst of air and water

Watch a video about floss-pick:

www.youtube.com/watch?v=BIYnSq9Yhrc

Watch a video about Water Floss:www.youtube.com/watch?v=kTQfwgl06gc

Watch a video about Air Floss

www.youtube.com/watch?v=EyZ81ijRtYI

Interdental Brushing: Another Addition to Flossing

If you want to go deeper in-between the teeth, then use an Interdental brush, particularly if you are unable to floss or if your gums have receded. It looks like a tiny bottle brush with bristles around a wire.

The use of an interdental brush is only advisable for people who have enough spaces in between teeth, which can happen if you have had surgery or recession due to some gum disease or gap due to the extraction of a tooth.

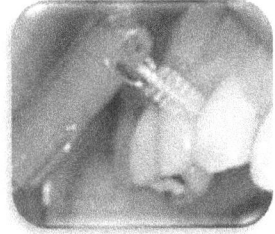

Watch a video about Interdental Brushing

www.youtube.com/watch?v=CYu3eq7x5Uw

www.youtube.com/watch?v=X7qrSmf4TYI&feature=related

Sulcabrush: Another Alternative to Interdental/ Subgingival Brushing

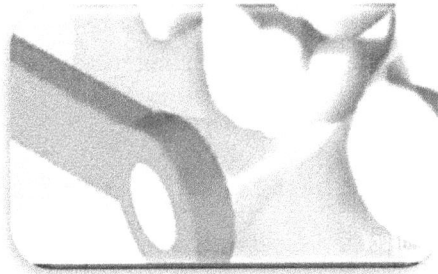

Squish the Sulcabrush against the inner or outer surface of the teeth and allow the bristles to follow the tooth surface right into the sulcus as you move the brush head toward the gumline. Sulca brushing is just like pushing cuticles except that the bristles go underneath the "cuticle" as it were. This is a bit counter-intuitive because it seems that you are pushing gunk into the sulcus. Perhaps you are! But it does not matter, as long as you follow the use of Sulcabrush with vigorous rinsing with water and then spitting. Plaque can only cause damage when it is organized into a biofilm that is capable of concentrating acids against the teeth and enzymes and other toxins against the gum (sulcus) lining. All that is needed is to disrupt (disorganize) the bacterial colony (biofilm) to stop this action and prevent the products from being concentrated. It takes about 24-36 hours for the biofilm to regrow and resume its action of concentrating toxins and acids. As an analogy think of scum growing on the surface of a stagnant pond. Stir it up with a stick and it will eventually regrow if left undisturbed.

Combine this technique once a day with an antiseptic such as an essential oil or colloidal liquid silver to control marginal gingivitis and gumline cavities.

Step 4: Do-It-Yourself (DIY) Scaling

Plaque is a sticky substance, full of bacteria, viruses, fungi and parasites. It builds on teeth. When plaque calcifies (hardens) over time, it is called tartar (in dental term called calculus).

- Plaque is the main cause of tooth decay and gum disease.
- You need to be aware of the fact that dental plaque is being formed continuously.

Scaling is the removal of calculus and plaque that attaches to the tooth surface, normally at the gumline and even below the gumline. A dental hygienist uses specific instruments and devices, such as a scaler to remove tartar.

Purpose

It is difficult to remove tartar by yourself, but you can remove freshly formed plaque if you remove it on a daily basis. Daily (better twice-a-day), proper removal will delay your next visit to the hygienist.

Tools

Use one of the following:

- The safest way to do DIY Scaling is to use the rubber tip, which you will find on the other end of many toothbrushes or use a rubber tip stimulator. Do not use metal scalers (hygienists are trained to use them).

- You may also use a toothpick fixed into a Perio-Aid handle.

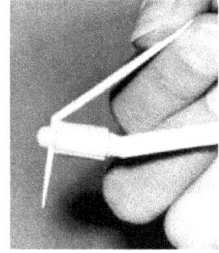

However, use of rubber tip is a preferred option.

Tasks

- Glide the tip of the rubber tip along the gumline, one tooth at a time, both inside and outside of both arches of teeth. Initially you may have to go back and forth on each tooth.

- Wipe or wash the rubber tip before cleaning a new surface.

- Rinse and swish with water to get rid of any food debris or plaque left in your mouth.

- Wash the tip with soap at the end of this step.

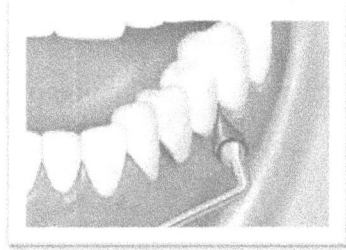

It is recommended to have a dental scaling by a dental hygienist, at 6 to 12 month intervals, depending how well you perform "DIY Scaling" regularly.

Since this step is remarkably similar to scaling, performed by a hygienist, we call this step "DIY Scaling".

Watch a video, about using a rubber tip

www.youtube.com/watch?v=Uxo5dvkKdJw&feature=related

Step 5: Final Brushing

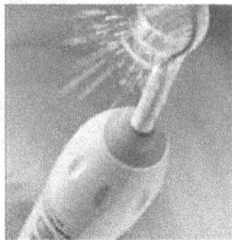

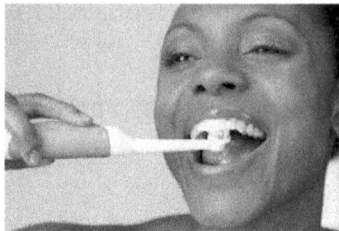

Electric Sonic Brush

Purpose

This is the second phase of brushing. No toothpaste is required, but if you have stained teeth then consider applying baking soda (or any other tooth powder). It is like massaging and polishing your teeth.

Tools

You will need an electric toothbrush (e.g. sonic vibration, see the image above). According to some research, electric toothbrushes remove 50% more plaque in comparison to manual brushes. You can adjust the pressure and vibrations with many of the electric brushes.

Tasks

With light pressure, you can start brushing from the gumline or below the gumline. Use the similar brushing technique described in Section 4 above for inner and outer surfaces of both dental arches.

Rinse with water or an organic mouthwash to remove any debris or bacteria that are still left on the teeth. You may use salt water as an effective disinfectant but not on a regular basis.

Step 6: Tongue Scraping

Purpose

Cleaning your tongue is crucial. Many pathogens are on the tongue and at the back of the tongue. Open your mouth and look in the mirror. You will see a layer of white deposit at the back of your tongue. Antibiotics and fungus infections make these white deposits worse. However, you should regularly scrape these white deposits off your tongue to reduce bacterial build-up. According to some dentists, you have more bacteria on the tongue than your gums (it is estimated that 80% of mouth bacteria reside on the tongue and cheeks), so it is equally if not more beneficial than some other steps. Food and pathogens left behind on your tongue can cause bad breath.

Tools

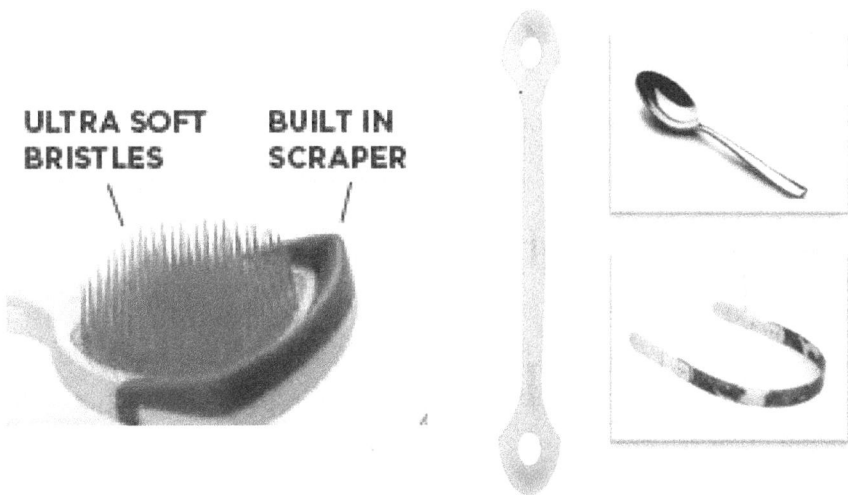

ULTRA SOFT BRISTLES   BUILT IN SCRAPER

You will need a tongue scraper (also called tongue cleaner).

Tongue scrapers come in various shapes and sizes.

- A small horseshoe shape metal or plastic device (see the image above)

- A flat plastic piece (see the image above)
- A small stainless steel teaspoon can also be used as a tongue scraper (see the image above)
- A combination of special soft brush for tongue and scraper (see the image above)
- Some toothbrushes have a rubber backing on the toothbrush head but these are not as effective as the other tongue scrapers mentioned above.

Tasks

- Starting from the back of the tongue, gently pull the white deposit forward and off your tongue. Go back as far as you can comfortably tolerate. Be gentle.

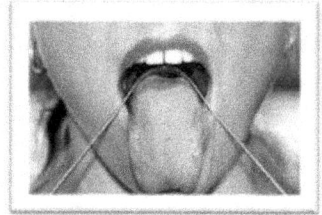

- Wash the scraper.
- Repeat three or four times, until the scraper is clean.
- Rinse your mouth.
- Wash the tongue scraper with soap when you finish.

Tip

Have you ever wondered why the tongue is whitish when you get up in the morning. Since there is minimal saliva flow during sleep, there is not enough saliva to neutralise the buildup of acid, bacteria or plaque, and it stays there as a white deposit. It is crucial to scrub your tongue in the morning before drinking or eating. Do scrape your tongue at bedtime again.

Step 7: Gum Massaging and Final Rinse

Purpose

Massage the gums to enhance circulation of blood to make them healthy. Previous steps such as brushing, flossing and tongue scraping were mechanical steps to remove food debris and bacteria. Now you also want to kill any leftover bacteria by rinsing with a mouthwash.

Tools

- Index Finger
- Mouthwash

Tasks

1. Gently massage your gums with your index finger using a circular motion.

2. Rinse your mouth with an antiseptic mouthwash. Swish and circulate the liquid.

3. Deep gargle: Retain and gargle the mouthwash as far as back in your throat you can.

4. Spit it out.

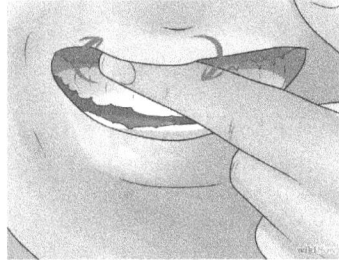

Section 5:
Oil Pulling for Healthy Gums

Oil Pulling is an Ayurvedic (ancient Indian) tradition of cleaning the mouth by using oil, which claims that not only does it kills bacteria in your mouth and gums but also cures (or prevents) many diseases. Oil Pulling is based on Ayurvedic life science that the tongue is mapped by organ-locations, that is, each section of the tongue is connected to all organs. It involves vigorously "chewing" two to three teaspoons (start with one) of Coconut oil for about 20 minutes (start with 10 minutes) and spitting it out.

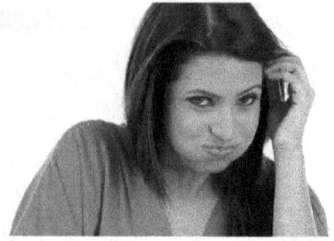

You can make this routine more effective by adding a drop or two of an essential oil, such as peppermint (open sinus), lemon (to detoxify), clove oil (relieve tooth pain) or oil of oregano (fight candida).

For more info, visit www.oilpulling.org

Section 6:
Weekly Dental
Hygiene Routine

In the above steps, we have discussed regular daily routines. This section will outline more dental hygiene routines which need to be performed on a weekly basis.

- Check the condition of your gums, teeth and inside of your mouth by using the dental mirror.

- Use disclosing tablets to examine the effectiveness of your brushing technique.

- Polish your teeth to remove any stains: You will need a natural tooth powder (two such powders are mentioned in the next section). Pour a little powder onto the palm of your clean dry hand, use it to rub onto the surfaces of your teeth. Rinse with water. Swish for 60 seconds before spitting out.

- If you have been using dental floss for interdental hygiene then use an alternate once a week, such as interdental brushes or water jet irrigator.

Tips about Toothbrushes and their Maintenance

Your toothbrush is loaded with germs, according to researchers at England's University of Manchester. They have found that one uncovered toothbrush can harbour more than 100 million bacteria, including *E. coli*, which can cause diarrhea, and staphylococci ("staph") bacteria that cause skin infections.

1. If you have a chronic problem, such as sore throat or cold, then sterilize your toothbrush or replace it every two weeks until you are healthy. Change your toothbrush again when you have recovered from illness.

2. Natural bristle brushes are more abrasive than nylon.

3. It is advisable to rotate two manual toothbrushes, giving enough time to dry the brush as it takes about 24 hours to dry. Bacteria breed in a moist environment. Dry toothbrushes by keeping its 'head up and handle down' in a glass or tumbler.

4. Sanitize your toothbrush, using a sanitizer or an antiseptic solution (explained in Section 6 of this chapter).

5. Keep your toothbrush away from the toilet (close the lid of your toilet when flushing).

6. Keep your toothbrush away from the toothbrushes of other people in your family.

7. Rinse your toothbrush thoroughly (preferably after applying a bit of soap).

Cleaning Toothbrushes and Other Dental Hygiene Tools

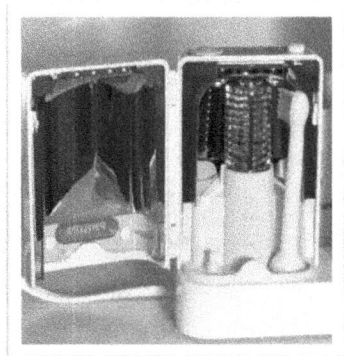

Every week (or whenever you are feeling sick) sterilize all brush heads of all toothbrushes, tip of the rubber tip stimulator. It is best to throw away dental floss and toothpicks after every use.

Sterilization

Use any of the following methods to sterilize (the process to kill germs using heat):

- Electric sterilizer that uses an ultraviolet lamp to sterilize the toothbrush. Some electric brush kits contain such a sterilizer. Some units have room for the brush head only and some you can use it for any type of toothbrush.
- High-heat dishwashing is the safest bet. Run your toothbrush through an automatic dishwasher, using HIGH heat to dry it.

Sanitization

Use the following solutions to kill the germs:

- Hydrogen peroxide 3% solution.
- An antiseptic mouthwash with essential oils (see the next section).

Submerge the bristles of your toothbrush (or any tools, such as tongue scraper, rubber tip stimulator) in one of the above solutions. Soak them for a minimum of 20 minutes or overnight, then remove and rinse the brush or tool and throw away the solution. Store the toothbrush (uncovered) upright in a container for air-drying.

Section 7:
Make Your Own Toothpaste and Mouthwash

If you cannot find non-toxic toothpaste and a mouthwash or you simply want to delve into making your own, then follow these simple recipes. If you enjoy cooking from scratch then you will love making your own dental products and save some money too. When you make your own dental products, you know the ingredients and their quality. You know that they do not contain any sugar (or sweeteners), fluorides or artificial flavours and best of all, no toxic ingredients (listed in Chapter 3).

Toothpaste

- Baking soda: 3 Tbsp.
- Salt: 1 Tbsp.
- Aloe Vera Gel: 3 Tbsp.
- Water: desired consistency or you may skip the water altogether.
- Add two to three drops of any essential oil e.g. peppermint, clove, or cinnamon oil.
- Optionally, use a little Xylitol for flavour ("tooth-friendly" sugar has anti-cavity properties).
- Optionally, use Calcium Bentonite Clay Powder or calcium powder or white Kaolin Clay: 2 Tbsp.

Baking soda and calcium can be abrasive if not finely powdered, so grind them fine in a coffee grinder. Mix all of the above ingredients before adding the water. Add the gel at the end.

Store in a sterilized, airtight container.

Tooth Powder

Modified Torrens Powder (MTP)

The original formula was published in the British Dental Journal about fifty years ago. It is based on remedies which have been with us since the beginning of time.

- 1 part salt
- 6 parts baking soda

Mix for five or more minutes in a grinder to make a fine powder. Store in a closed container.

How to Use Tooth powder to fight gum disease:

- Wash your hands. Dip your index finger in 1½% hydrogen peroxide.
- Dip the wet finger into the powder and onto the gums (inside and outside).
- Rinse your mouth.

This is a morning and not at night routine. It tonifies the gums and helps prevent infections.

Mouthwashes

Mouthwash is as important as the toothpaste; it rinses your teeth, tongue and mouth, gets rid of any food debris floating in your mouth, and eliminates any odour. Baking soda combined with Essential oils makes a soothing and antiseptic mouthwash. You may also find them helpful when fighting a sore throat and cold.

Essential Oil Based Mouthwash (preferred)

- Half a teaspoon of baking soda.
- Half a glass of water.
- Two to three drops of peppermint oil.
- Two to three drops of clove oil (it has anti-fungal, anti-viral and antiseptic properties).
- Two to three drops of thyme (one of the strongest antiseptics).

Hydrogen Peroxide Based Mouthwash

As a variation, you can make a mouthwash with 3% hydrogen peroxide with an equal quantity of water (half-and-half). Do not use this if you have any metal restorations (such as mercury amalgam) in your mouth.

Mouthwash from Modified Torrens Powder (MTP)

Three tsp of MTP (explained above) mixed with 6 oz. of hot water.

It is better to make mouthwash when you need it but if you wish, you can make a large enough quantity for a few days. Store in a sterilized airtight container.

Saturated saline is also recommended as a better mouthwash.

Section 8:
Conclusions

It is not necessary to perform all the steps every time, but do all of the seven-steps before you go to sleep. I do steps 1 and 2 after breakfast, and the entire program regularly after lunch and after supper. I prefer to floss my teeth before brushing them, particularly after eating fibre rich food such as an orange and a pineapple. If you want to reduce your acidity and pathogens, then rinse your mouth before eating any meal (or at least drink a little water).

> If you take stain-causing foods (such as coffee, tea, wine, blueberries, etc.) then rinse immediately. Drink a little water if you are unable to rinse. In general drinking water increases saliva production. This helps in removing pathogens and reduces the acidity in the mouth.
>
> Eating a little hard cheese after a meal is also good for your teeth due to calcium and phosphorus in the cheese; the salt in the cheese reduces acidity too.

Remember to wash your hands every time you brush your teeth, both before and after, to prevent the transfer of germs.

If you are dreading a visit to the dentist, then following the above procedures will reduce your fear. Think of protecting your teeth from decay, gums from infection and your nerves from a close encounter with the dentist's drill.

It is my belief that there is no part of the body that cannot be cleaned easily but when it comes to teeth, it is a challenge. It appears that nature has conspired with dentists to keep them busy.

OK, I will modify my statement - We may not have the best design of teeth *for the kind of foods and lifestyle we are using today.*

Yes, there are still traditional cultures in some parts of Africa and Asia where people have kept healthy teeth for their lifetime because they have not been exposed to a Western diet. In the meantime, I will stick to my theory: We do not have the best design when it comes to teeth!

CHAPTER 5

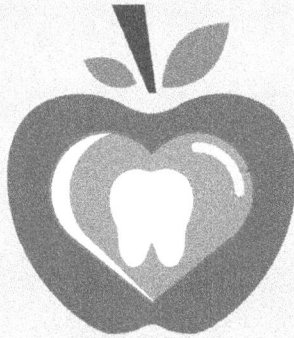

Ingredients of
Tooth Care Products

Klaus Ferlow and Max Haroon

Effort is like toothpaste: you can usually
squeeze out just a little bit more.
~Author Unknown

There are thousands of dental care products on the market today, ranging from daily use consumer products, such as toothpastes and mouthwashes, to occasional use dental products such as tooth whiteners and oral irrigators.

This chapter examines the ingredients used in commercially available products so that you can make an informed decision on whether they are as good as they claim.

Fluoride toothpaste has not only received the seal of approval from all Dental Authorities, but according to them, it is necessary for preventive dental care. However, our opinion differs and if you research with an open mind, we are sure you will agree with us.

Section 1:
The Truth About
Commercial Toothpastes

Modern toothpaste is a heavy mix of chemicals and synthetics meant to clean, polish and maintain healthy teeth and gums. Are those ingredients safe or even necessary?

Have you given any thought to what you are swishing around your mouth at least twice a day?

One of the fastest ways to absorb anything into the body is through the mouth. Because of this, you should be aware that potentially harmful toxic ingredients in your toothpaste and mouthwash could also be absorbed into your body.

It seems that toothpaste is almost as old as teeth, and ancient populations used abrasives, such as crushed oyster shells, bone and eggshells mixed with flavouring and powdered charcoal. Later essential oils made from peppermint, spearmint or cinnamon, made brushing more pleasant and helped kill bacteria and germs at the same time.

Common brand toothpastes contain large sized abrasive particles that can quickly wear away tooth enamel. The body does not regenerate tooth enamel; its loss is permanent and can never be replaced. As tooth enamel is lost, the softer dentin material underneath is exposed and thereby significantly enhances the risk of dental decay and tooth loss.

Most commercial toothpastes (including Specialty toothpastes for enamel protection and sensitivity) contain ingredients such as SLS (sodium lauryl sulphate), fluoride, sodium laureth sulphate, sodium saccharin, artificial colour & scent (flavour), some even contain sugar.

Children toothpaste often has flavours, which taste like candy or bubble gum that may tempt them to swallow it. This can be a problem, and the US government requires the following warning label to be provided on toothpastes:

> "Keep out of reach of children under 6 years of age. If you accidentally swallow more than used for brushing, seek professional assistance or contact the Poison Control Center immediately. As with other toothpastes, if irritation occurs discontinue use".

Did it ever cross your mind why manufacturers of commercial toothpaste have to give this "warning" on the labels?

Direction to Use Toothpaste

Adults and children over 6 years:

Apply pea size amount of toothpaste onto soft bristle toothbrush. Brush thoroughly after meals or at least twice a day; follow our Seven Steps Protocol, outlined in the Chapter 2.

Children between 2 to 6 years:

To minimize swallowing, use smaller than a pea size amount and supervise brushing until correct habits are established. Even better, replace the toothpaste with Aloe Vera Gel.

Children under 2 years:

Children under 2 years should never use toothpaste: ask a dentist or doctor for advice.

Toothpaste Ingredients

Many types of commercially available toothpastes contain one or more of the following ingredients (mostly harmful) shown in the Table 1 and Table 2 below. These ingredients are also found in many other skin care and personal care products such as mouthwashes and shampoos.

Analysis of toothpaste ingredients is a challenging task because many manufacturers do not disclose all ingredients and their exact proportions (proprietary protection).

Commercial toothpastes contain the following categories of ingredients. Each Ingredient can be an Active or Inactive, depending on its function in the toothpaste. The Active ingredients are for the health and hygiene (cleaning) of teeth while Inactive are added to formulate the toothpaste as a product, such as favour, colour, binding, moisturising.

#	Category	Function
	Table 1	
	Categories of Ingredients used in Toothpastes	
1	Abrasive ingredients	To abrade enamel and remove food stains
2	Polishing ingredients	To polish rough surfaces
3	Bleaching ingredients	To make teeth whiter
4	*Moisturisers	To stop the toothpaste becoming dry
5	*Binders & Surfactants	To hold all the ingredients together
6	*Foaming & Detergent	To degrease food particles like soap and also generates foam
7	*Colours	To make toothpaste look pretty
8	*Flavours & Sweeteners	To taste yummy
9	*Preservatives	To increase the shelf life of toothpaste
10	*Water	To increase its volume
11	Antibacterial	To fight decay and to kill germs

* Inactive Ingredients

© Max Haroon 2012

The table below provides estimated proportion of various commonly used ingredients in toothpastes under eleven categories.

#	Category	% of total Tooth-paste	Commonly used Ingredients
		Table 2: Ingredients (toxic & non-toxic)	
1 & 2	Abrasive & Polishing	50% approx.	Alumina trihydrate, Calcium carbonate (abrasive), calcium pyrophosphate, Dihydrate dicalcium phosphate, *Hydrated Silica, magnesium trisilicate, Pumice (abrasive), silica gels, sodium metaphosphate, Zirconium silicate (abrasive)
3	Bleaching & Whiteners		Sodium carbonate peroxide
4	Moisturisers	25% approx.	*Diethylene glycol (DEG), glycerol, *propylene glycol, *sodium lauryl sulphate (SLS), sorbitol
5	Binders & Surfactants		Natural gums: Arabic, karaya and tragacanth, the seaweed colloids (alginates, Irish moss extract and gum carrageenan) Synthetic cellulose: Carboxymethyl cellulose, hydroxyethyl cellulose, *sodium lauryl sulphate
6	Foaming & Detergent		Lauryl sarcosinate, *sodium lauryl sulphate (SLS), *sodium fluoride
7	Colours		*FD & C Blue No. 1 & 2
8	Flavours & Sweeteners		*Sodium saccharin Natural – Mostly from Essential Oils: anise, caraway, cinnamon, citrus, clove, eucalyptus, menthol, nutmeg, peppermint, pimento, spearmint, thyme, wintergreen
9	Preservatives		*Parabens
10	Water	25% approx.	
11	Antibacterial		*Sodium fluoride, *triclosan, +neem, Essential oils

*Toxic ingredients described in Section 2

Some Non-toxic ingredients are described in Section 3

© Max Haroon 2012

Section 2:
Toxic Ingredients

There are a large number of toothpastes available on the market, and the vast majority contain a variety of different harmful ingredients.

One of the purpose of the book is to reiterate the message '**read the ingredients label**' when you are buying herbal, medicinal, personal care or any product.

People just have to make some effort to find out about herbal products that do not use dangerous, hazardous chemicals, synthetics, artificial colours or flavours.

Some toxic ingredients listed and marked with * in the above table are described below alphabetically. Some non-toxic ingredients are described in Section 3.

Diethylene Glycol (DEG) DEG is a non-ionic surfactant used in shampoo, **toothpaste** and cleansing preparations. Ethylene glycol groups are carcinogenic, mutagenic, causing adverse reactions or are toxic, absorb through the skin, and are hazardous if used on large areas of the body; ingestion can be fatal.

FD & C Blue No. 1 & 2

These artificial colourings/dyes are often found in familiar toothpaste brands plus a wide variety of other products. Recent studies indicate that they can trigger a large number of behavioural, comprehension and health issues, and they may cause severe allergic and other reactions such as asthma, headaches, nausea, fatigue, nervousness and cancer. They are derived from crude oil, synthesized from petroleum. These dyes may be absorbed within seconds through the skin on the lips, or the mouth. The mucosal lining inside of the mouth has an absorption efficiency of more than 91% and these carcinogens get into your blood, your brain, and your cells in no time at all, especially when you consider most people use dental care products two to three times a day!

Often used to colour toothpastes blue, most coal tar derivatives are potential carcinogens, cause allergic reactions, teratogen or toxic and have been known to produce malignant tumours at the site of injection and by ingestion in rats.

Hydrated Silica

Made from a crystallized compound found in quartz, sand and flint. Used as an abrasive and tooth whitener which damages the tooth-enamel. Enamel remineralizes from the ionic calcium and phosphorus in the saliva. Scratching the surface of the tooth with an abrasive like hydrated silica harms the enamel and prevents remineralisation, much like using sand to clean glass. Severe wear may eventually occur. While this ingredient could abrogate tartar and make teeth whiter, they might also do harm to dental health by altering the alkaline/acidic balance of the mouth, gums and tongue. Health hazards from chemicals and toxins in our oral hygiene products are the most circumventable of all the health hazards we face.

Propylene Glycol (PG)

Petrochemical absorbs quickly into the skin and irritates it. It is used in many personal care products as humectants (moisturizer), surfactants, solvents and even in anti-freeze. It has been shown to cause liver abnormalities and kidney damage in laboratory animals. It may cause allergic reactions, acne, and contact dermatitis.

Sodium Lauryl Sulphate (SLS)

This is a detergent, humectant, emulsifier and foaming agent. Do not be deceived if it says on the label "derived from coconut!" It is a combination of lauryl alcohol and mineral sodium sulphate, followed by neutralization with sodium carbonate. SLS is also found in car wash soap, engine degreasers, garage floor cleaners, shampoos, and shaving foams. It can degenerate cell membranes, alter the genetic information in cells (mutagenic) and can damage the immune system. It is reported to cause eye irritation, skin rashes, hair loss, dandruff, allergic reactions and canker sores. It penetrates into your eyes, brain and liver and can stay there for a long time.

Sodium Laureth Sulphate (SLES)

To make SLS less irritating, it is often ethoxylated (by adding ethylene oxide), resulting in the modified compound of SLES. But SLES is also a concern because it can be contaminated with 1,4-dioxane, which may cause cancer (according to the International Agency for Research on Cancer), and it stays in the environment for a long time. Contamination occurs during the process of ethoxylation.

Sodium Fluoride

It is derived from hydrofluoric, made by reacting sulphuric acid with fluorspar, an ore rich calcium fluoride, a hazardous chemical. Did you know that fluoride is the main ingredient in rat poison?

Despite fluoride being prescribed by doctors for over 50 years, the US Food and Drug Administration (FDA) have never approved any fluoride product designed for ingestion as safe or effective, since fluoride is a cumulative poison. Additionally, a 1991 study stated that fluoride has been shown NOT to reduce cavities and scientists are linking it to dental fluorosis, arthritis, allergic reactions and about ten thousand preventable deaths every year from cancer (from fluoride and ambiguous carcinogens, Federal Cancer Institute).

On average, only 50% of the fluoride we ingest each day is excreted through the kidneys. The remainder accumulates in our bones, pineal gland, and other tissues. Fluoride will accumulate in the kidney, if the kidney is malfunctioning or is damaged, it will increase an individual's susceptibility to fluoride poisoning.

www.fluoridealert.org/health/kidney/

Researchers have linked fluoride to thyroid cancer, but no one is listening! Fluoride is especially dangerous for young children who tend to swallow it after brushing their teeth. Many types of toothpaste contain enough fluoride in a 120 ml. (4 oz.) tube to poison a young child.

On some labels, it says, *"If a large amount is swallowed, call poison control centre"*! That is why many toothpaste manufacturers include a warning on their labels, *"Not for use by children under the age of 6 years"*.

Fluoride can corrode the tooth enamel and when swallowed can lead to Crohn's disease. Fluoride does not reduce cavities and scientists are linking it to dental deformity, arthritis and allergic reactions.

According to the following referenced article: Fluorosis (excessive exposure to high concentration of fluoride) can result in darkened or mottled teeth, erosion of enamel, compromised bone structure and a lot of other problems including learning disabilities, kidney disease and brain lesions.

Read the article "Hidden Fluoride in Our Food"

truthtalk13.wordpress.com/2013/07/23/hidden-fluoride-in-our-food/

In the interest of informed consent, please pursue the following links presenting opposing viewpoints regarding the use of fluoride:

Policy Statement of the Royal College of Dental Surgeons of Ontario
rcdso.org/assets/documents/dispatch/dispatch_2003_v17_no2.pdf

The Fluoride Deception - an interview with Christopher Bryson
fluoridealert.org/fan-tv/bryson/

Fluoridation of Water

Fluoride is added to water in an attempt to prevent tooth decay. We oppose this practice by municipal authorities for the following reasons:

1.   According to the National Academy of Sciences, fluoride is not an essential nutrient. The human body does not need fluoride for any physiological process.

2.   Most dental researchers now concede that fluoride's main benefit comes from direct contact with the outside of teeth (a "topical" effect), and not from ingestion (a "systemic" effect). There is no need to swallow fluoride to prevent tooth decay.

3.   The main fluoride chemical added to water (hydrofluorosilicic acid) is an industrial by-product from the phosphate fertilizer industry. It is an unpurified, industrial-grade, corrosive acid which has been linked, in several recent studies, to increased levels of lead in children's blood.

4.   Recent studies in the peer-reviewed medical literature indicate that fluoridated water can have detrimental side effects. Health risks associated with low-to-moderate doses of fluoride include: dental fluorosis, bone fracture, bone cancer, joint pain, skin rash, reduced thyroid activity, and IQ deficits.

For more info, visit cof-cof.ca/

Sodium Saccharin

Sodium saccharin is an artificial sweetener and can cause mutagenic, toxic or adverse reactions. Tests on rats in the 1980's developed bladder cancer. The FDA (Federal Drug Administration, USA) also lists it as a possible carcinogen. It is currently being evaluated by the National Toxicology Program.

Triclosan

Used as an antimicrobial to prevent the growth of harmful bacteria. It is also called an antibacterial, antivirus and antifungal and is used in a large variety of household goods and personal care products. Some such products are liquid hand soaps, **toothpaste,** deodorants, processed food, clothing, dish soap, detergent, floor wash, disinfecting sprays, glass cleaners, mouthwash, laundry soaps, lotions, moisturizers, children's toys and cleaning supplies.

"... Further, some data suggest that long-term exposure to certain active ingredients used in antibacterial products—for example, triclosan (liquid soaps) and triclocarban (bar soaps) —could pose health risks, such as bacterial resistance or hormonal effects". FDA Statement January 24, 2014

Studies at the Institute of Odontology in Huddingen, Sweden, the Virginia Tech University in Blacksburg, USA and the University of Victoria, Canada have shown that triclosan may promote the emergence of bacteria that are resistant to antibiotics, may develop allergies and asthma in children, and may interfere with thyroid hormones. It is a health hazard to humans, as well as wildlife. The American Medical Association suggests that consumers should check the product ingredient lists for triclosan, tricocarban, quaternary ammonium and microban. It is a suspected carcinogen. More www.health-report.co.uk/triclosan.html

> "... in the environment, it pollutes water and then transforms into something much worse, the cancer-causing agent dioxin. Three-quarters of North American have triclosan residues in in their urine; it is even common in breast milk".
>
> Dr. Mike Roizen and Dr. Mehmet Oz, writing about Triclosan.

These are just a few key chemical ingredients you will find in many types of toothpaste, but there are other harmful ingredients found in toothpastes that are hazardous to your health. Therefore, **Read Carefully All Ingredients On The Labels**. If you cannot pronounce the name of an ingredient, it is most likely a harmful chemical and you should not buy it!

Here, is what most people do not know about harmful chemicals in personal care products:

Nobody can be entirely sure that all manufacturers list all ingredients: medicinal, non-medicinal, toxic or non-toxic, on the label.

If a product lists a number of herbal extracts and several chemical ingredients, nobody knows what the percentages are of the ingredients or how effective are those small dosages. For example, if you use between 0.01% - 0.05% of herbal extracts, it does not mean that all herbal extracts are effective, since the dosage is far too low. When, at the same time, a number of toxic and synthetic chemicals are listed, they work synergistically together as a unit, instantly killing the herbal extracts and even turning the product poisonous. When companies list SLS (sodium lauryl sulphate) as an ingredient and in parenthesis indicate "derived from coconut", people are deceived into thinking this is a natural product.

Since large corporations cannot afford to have an herbal product go bad (e.g. rancid), they add a variety of chemical preservatives (mostly parabens), which prevents spoilage of the product on the retail shelf. These products can sometimes last for many years on the store shelves. Recalls of large quantities of products are very costly and will kill the sale of the product and give the company a poor reputation.

One of the fastest ways to absorb anything into the body is through the mouth. Your daily routine of brushing your teeth with your favourite toothpaste may also be delivering a daily dose of antibiotics or other potentially toxic ingredients, without you realizing it.

There are very few types of toothpaste that are "almost" chemical-free, but you have to do your own research.

Section 3:
Nontoxic Ingredients

Here are some non-toxic ingredients, used as a cure for dental conditions and natural toothpastes.

Baking Soda (Sodium Bicarbonate)

Baking soda is the main rising agent in baking powder. It has a history in cleaning teeth; it was used in tooth powders around the 18th century. Towards the end of the 19th century, tooth powders were mass-produced using baking soda. Baking soda is alkaline (refer to chapter 11 for discussion of alkaline and acidity) and it neutralizes acidity of the mouth and kills bacteria. A solution of baking soda (small amount dissolved in water) is an excellent substitute if you cannot find a natural/nontoxic- toothpaste. You can also make your own toothpaste using baking soda, read Chapter 2 for the details.

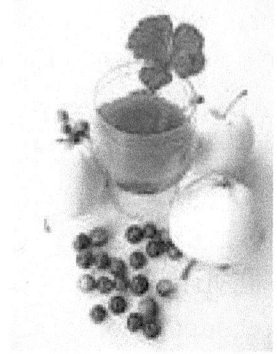

Cranberry

A team led by oral biologist **Hyun (Michel) Koo, D.D.S., Ph.D.,** at the University of Rochester Medical Center has discovered that the same traits that make cranberry juice a powerful weapon against bladder infections also hold promise for protecting teeth against cavities. Koo found that cranberry juice acts like Teflon® for teeth, making it difficult for the bacteria to cling to tooth surfaces. Stickiness is everything for the microbe *Streptococcus mutans,* which creates most cavities by eating sugars and then excreting acids that cause dental decay.

The Neem (Azadirachta indica)

Neem is native to India and has been a key ingredient in Ayurvedic formulations for more than 5000 years, one of the world's oldest healing science systems. Neem is affectionately known as the "Village Pharmacy" and as "Sarva Roga Nivarin" (healer of all ailments). Although almost all parts of the neem tree are used medicinally, oil derived

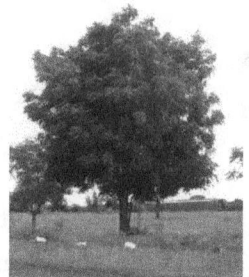

from the seeds and extracts from the leaves are used more frequently in modern applications. Neem is used to treat skin diseases (including acne, eczema, and psoriasis), to improve oral hygiene, to reduce fevers, to expel worms and to fight infections. In addition, neem demonstrates a natural ability to repel a wide variety of insects, prevent sunburns and is an anti-malarial medication.

It is only recently that the rest of the world has started to show interest in and recognize neem's healing potential. Of all the powerful healing plants throughout the ages, few offer such value and versatility as the neem tree. With its increasing popularity, it is obvious that this ancient miracle is also effective for the ailments of a modern world.

More information about the neem

www.positivehealth.com/article/herbal-medicine/neem-true-botanical-panacea

*Source: **Neem: Nature's Healing Gift to Humanity***, Klaus Ferlow

Peelu Tree (Salvadoran Persica Arak)

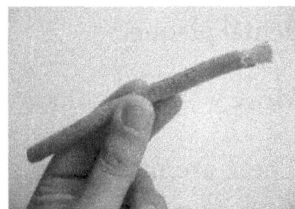

The Peelu Tree is known by many names throughout the world: Miswak and Siwak. Whichever name you choose, the twigs and fibres of this Middle Eastern tree have been used since the time of the Prophet Muhammad, who is said to have recommended its use to clean teeth and the mouth.

Use of Peelu twig dates back to the middle of the first millennia, it is believed that the "Kayu Sugi", or chewing stick, is the world's oldest toothbrush. Traditionally, the outer bark is removed and a person chews on the interior fibres for gentle, nonabrasive oral care. Today, science is proving the effectiveness of this ancient dental health tool. All-natural Peelu products provide a healthy way to enjoy fresh breath, as well as healthy gums and teeth, without artificial chemicals, toxins or abrasives. **For more information about Peelu:** www.peelu.com/about-us.html

Mastic (Pistacia Lentiscus)

The mastic tree is native to the Mediterranean regions of Greece. It was not until Iraqi researchers published a study in 1984 that mastic received international attention. Their research demonstrated that chewing mastic gum was an effective means for reducing dental plaque. Other researchers quickly jumped on the bandwagon and proclaimed the benefit of mastic in eliminating bacteria, not only from the mouth but also from the digestive tract. Now there is growing scientific evidence to support the use of mastic for reducing the risk of tooth decay and improving gastric health.

The best way to look after your teeth is to brush and floss right after every meal - but that is often impractical. Alternatively, you can rinse your mouth thoroughly with water or an antibacterial mouthwash after eating, or drink green tea, which has antibacterial properties, or chew gum (made from mastic) for about ten minutes after each meal. Chewing sugar-free mastic gum after a meal reduces the acidity of dental plaque.

More www.life-enhancement.com/article_template.asp?ID=662

There are many brands of natural toothpastes but do check out the ingredients in spite of their claim to be natural toothpastes.

More non-toxic ingredients are described in Chapter 4.

Section 4:
A Word About Mouthwash

Most people use mouthwash to eliminate bad breath caused by food stuck between the teeth and bacteria, which feed off this accumulation of food. However, experts say that mouthwash does not live up to its reputation. It works only for a short time by killing lots of germs. Nevertheless, this is followed by the high alcohol content drying your mouth. Bacteria cannot be washed away when the mouth is dry, so it flourishes and causes even more bad breath.

Mouthwash may make your breath smell better for a short period, but what have you done to your immune system, oesophagus and stomach lining? In addition, what about that chemical soup your liver is required to detoxify? Do you really need to add more chemicals to your already toxic overload of your body? In a study done at the Division of Restorative Dentistry in Bristol, UK, researchers found that the use of acidic (low pH) mouthwash causes erosion of dental enamel that is directly correlated to the sensitivity in teeth. People complain with less enamel of much greater tooth sensitivity to hot and cold. Think about it before you purchase the next bottle of mouthwash and if you do check the ingredients on the label.

Could there be any correlation between the use of "chemical" mouthwash and an epidemic known as acid reflux disease? Daily use of mouthwash has been linked to increased incidents of oral cancer, erosion of the tooth enamel, increased tooth sensitivity and higher risks of bad breath according to recent studies from the University of Sao Paulo, Brazil. Results indicated that daily mouthwash use was strongly associated with cancer of the pharynx (serves both the respiratory system and the digestive system receiving air from the nasal cavity and air, food and water from the oral cavity) and with cancer of the mouth. In another study, at the Division of Restorative Dentistry in Bristol, UK, researchers found that the use of low pH (acidic) mouthwashes cause erosion of dental enamel that is directly correlated to sensitivity in teeth. Low pH indicates acidity and most popular mouthwashes sold at traditional retail outlets are highly acidic. For example, Listerine has a pH of 4.3, Scope has a pH of 5.0, and neutral pH level is 7.0 with declining values increased levels of acidity. Healthy body saliva has a pH between 6.4 – 6.8.

If someone has bad breath (most often caused by a gum infection), has to change their diet from junk food and soda drinks to quality nutritional food, quit smoking and limit alcohol use. Your body's natural line of defense against bacteria is your saliva that is rich in oxygen as well as other critical enzymes needed to eliminate unwanted bacteria in the mouth.

Individuals who eat a lot of garlic can eat parsley and drink a glass of water or use aspartame free peppermint or eucalyptus candy or sugar-free chewing gum.

You have to explore for yourself if any mouthwashes are available without harmful ingredients.

Section 5:
Tooth Whiteners,
Should They Be Avoided?

Everybody wants a sparkling smile. But, do tooth whiteners really work? Are they harmless to your teeth and gums?

It is no secret that healthy white teeth can help enhance your appearance and boost your overall self-confidence, and for the most part, people define "healthy teeth" as bright, white, and stain-free. Did you know that teeth whitening is the number one most requested cosmetic procedure in North America? This trend does not show any sign of slowing down.

 People have been able to take advantage of professional whitening services from their dentist for many years now. Today, you can find whitening strips, gels, trays, and lights anywhere from your dentist office to your local health and grocery store, pharmacy, etc. They are quick, easy to use, and can be effective at removing unsightly stains and brightening up your teeth.

Perfect, right? Not really!

Most of these products contain some type of peroxide to remove stains. In some cases, the hydrogen peroxide, along with a variety of other chemicals found in these products, can cause alarming problems such as gum irritation and tooth sensitivity.

Overuse of at-home whitening kits has some serious risks. Not only can they cause sensitivity, they can also damage tissues and wear the enamel down so much that your teeth look almost see-through and very unnatural. Eventually, they can become odd shades of blue and grey.

The off-white colour of teeth that most people find unsightly and unattractive is the colour that your teeth are **meant** to look, unless it is caused by stains.

We still do not know any of the long-term side effects of using bleaching products. If you would like to get a more dazzling smile, why not try some natural alternatives:

- **Baking soda**: put a little bit on your toothbrush with your toothpaste.
- **Crunchy vegetables**: celery, carrots, broccoli, and cucumbers are natural abrasives and can help scrub away stains.

Remember, if you do not have healthy teeth, you are not a healthy person either.

Section 6:
Effect of Toxic Ingredients

Most of the ingredients are not approved by FDA, some toxic ingredients are even registered with EPA and others as pesticide, or possible carcinogen (agent causing cancer) but still used by the cosmetic industry. Here Are few ill-effects:

1. Degenerate cell membrane.

2. Mutagenic: Alter genetic information in cells (undesirable mutation may also occur in some later generation)

3. Damage immune system

4. Some are hormones disruptors.

5. Produces an unwanted effect when the chemical has reached a sufficient concentration at a certain part of the body.

Cosmetic and body care industry is highly unregulated, no pre-product approval Are required. A basic approval process exists for color additives.

For more information about toxic ingredients:

http://life-transformation-institute.org/health/index.htm

CHAPTER 6

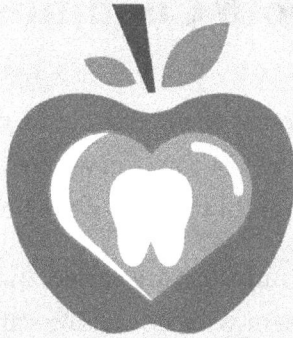

Common Tooth Conditions and Their Remedies

Klaus Ferlow

Tooth decay was a perennial national problem that meant a
mouthful of silver for patients, and for dentists a pocketful of gold
~ Claudia Wallis

Section 1:
Tooth Conditions

Tooth conditions are almost as severe and as varied as the rest of the body's illnesses, and that may be a reason why we have two sets of doctors - one for teeth and another for the rest of the body!

Symptoms for various conditions are varied, but the underlying causes are the same: they all begin with not taking care of your teeth both in cleaning them and in nourishing them.

Therefore, prevention mentioned in any of the following conditions (given alphabetically) will apply to all conditions of the body. This book outlines holistic health of the entire body, so it is advised that you follow the entire book.

- Bad Breath and Tongue
- Gingivitis
- Gum Bleeding
- Loose Tooth
- Periodontal Disease
- Pyorrhoea
- Root Canal
- Teething in Infants
- Tooth Grinding (Bruxism)
- Tooth Sensitivity
- Tooth Stains
- Toothache and Tooth Decay

- Wisdom Teeth

Bad Breath and Tongue

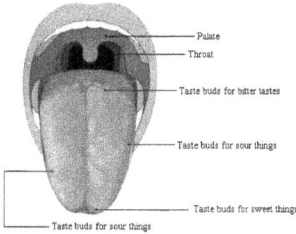

Palate
Throat
Taste buds for bitter tastes
Taste buds for sour things
Taste buds for sweet things
Taste buds for sour things

The tongue is widely used by many holistic traditions, especially in the Traditional Chinese and Ayurveda medicine, as an indicator of the overall health of the body as well as organs. The tissue of the tongue is a continuation of the stomach and digestive system, so the tongue is a reliable indication of the condition of the digestive organs.

Symptoms

- A pale, flaccid tongue indicates weakness, anaemia, and a tendency toward fluid retention.

- A deep red tongue indicates an inflammation condition.

- A white-coated tongue represents an overly alkaline state with coldness, poor digestion, and internal congestion of the digestive system and/or the lungs.

- A yellow-coated tongue signifies an overly acid state, toxicity, inflammation, and congestion.

- A red coloured tongue, heavily fissured and smooth, lacking normal papillae or small whitish bumps, is a certain indication of B-complex deficiency.

- A trembling tongue indicates general weakness of the nervous system.

- A stiff, rigid tongue indicates tenseness, while a tongue with tooth marks on the edge tells of fluid retention, possibly low energy and over-laxness. This is called scalloping of the tongue.

Causes

Bad breath is a combination of unhealthy diet and odour originating from the stomach and tongue. The tongue is covered with microscopic, hair-like projections that trap and harbour plaque and food.

Halitosis causes are often the result of eating or drinking a product that causes odour to escape from the mouth. Most people experience halitosis causes from foods like garlic and onions, but there are many other products that are also halitosis causes. Many of these products do not smell particularly bad before being ingested. Food items that are known to be halitosis causes include fish, cheese, and acidic beverages like coffee.

From www.webmd.com

Remedy

A daily gentle scrubbing of tongue, including the top of the tongue. You will see the added benefit if cleaning is done as the first task when you get up in the morning to get rid of any plaque deposit while you were sleeping. A large number of people suffer from silent acid reflux (they are not aware); a white coated tongue after getting up is an indicator of this acid reflux or of poor brushing technique at bedtime.

Gingivitis

Symptoms

Gingivitis is classified as an inflammation of the gums which when untreated can lead to a serious gum disease. Early signs of gingivitis are bleeding, dark red or purple, swollen and tender gums. Mouth sores also indicate gingivitis.

If gingivitis is not treated in time, it will create several other infections and conditions including tooth loss, jaw abscess, trench mouth, gum abscess and infection and periodontitis.

Causes

- Gingivitis is caused by bacteria build-up. There is a constant build-up of both good and bad bacteria in your mouth, depending on your hygiene. Bad bacteria cause plaque build-up. The combination of plaque and tartar continue to inflame the gums which can develop into gingivitis.

- Commercial toothpaste and mouthwash contain harmful chemical ingredients that worsen bacterial problems in the mouth. These ingredients dehydrate your mouth and irritate your gums. In some extreme cases they can even set the stage for bacteria formation in the mouth.

Gum Bleeding

You should be seriously concerned when you have bleeding gums. It is a precursor to gingivitis or it can be a symptom of gingivitis (inflammation of the gum tissues). Bleeding and gingivitis are connected with further health problems.

Causes

- Improper oral hygiene
- Hormonal changes in women
- Cancer and chemotherapy

Remedies

- Avoid food with sharp edges like peanuts, potato chips or tacos.
- Use soft bristle brushes and brush carefully to avoid banging the toothbrush into your gums.
- Do not use tobacco products.
- Be careful about extremely hot or cold foods and drinks.
- Use chemical-free herbal toothpaste to brush your teeth; it works just after using it for few times.
- Wet a black tea bag in warm water and apply it to the gums.

- Sprinkle white concentrated stevia powder on top of toothpaste on the toothbrush. Gently massage the gums in circular motions.
- Gargle with stevia (1/2 glass warm water with ¼ tsp stevia) to alleviate painful gums, sore throat and mouth sores.

Loose Teeth

Hold warm apple cider vinegar in your mouth and spit it out, repeat several times a day. You can also use boiled sage with honey (after cooling the solution). Brush tooth with baking soda.

Periodontal Disease

Periodontal disease or periodontitis is the advanced stage of gingivitis. Many people have lost their teeth, including some young people due to this disease.

Periodontal disease is second only to the common cold as the most prevalent disease in North America. It is the major cause of tooth loss, especially in adults. The rate of periodontal disease increases with age, ranging from 15% at age ten to more than 50% at age fifty. Periodontal means "located around the tooth".

Causes

Gingivitis is the early stage of periodontal disease caused by breathing through the mouth, badly fitting fillings and prostheses that irritate the surrounding gum tissue, and a diet consisting of too many soft

foods that rob the teeth and gums of much needed "exercise". Smokers are more susceptible than non-smokers to periodontitis and tooth loss. Periodontal disease can be made worse by missing teeth, food impaction, malocclusion, tongue thrusting, teeth grinding and toothbrush trauma.

Bleeding gums may signal a vitamin C deficiency. Dryness and cracking at the corner of the mouth may indicate a deficiency of vitamin B2 (riboflavin).

Symptoms

Periodontitis is often a silent disease as those who suffer from it rarely experience pain, and may not even be aware that there is a problem. Some indications are gums pulling away from the teeth, loose teeth, space developing between the teeth, persistent bad taste, pus between teeth and gums, tender gums when touched, swollen, inflamed and receding gums, bright red and purple gums, tooth loss and bad breath.

Effect

It is estimated that 85% of the population have some form of gum disease. The truth is that although periodontal disease may originate in the mouth, it can affect the entire body and increasing the risk of several other adverse health effects including:

- Increased risk of heart attacks by up to 25%
- Respiratory disease
- Digestive disorders
- Increased risk of stroke by a factor of 10
- Pancreatic cancer
- Problems controlling both type I and type II diabetes

Problems in the mouth often are reflections of deficiencies or underlying disorders of the body.

A recent study showed that the medical cost of those with periodontal diseases was 21% higher than those without it.

Periodontitis is not something to be taken lightly. Seek professional help immediately. Remember, if you do not have healthy teeth, you do not have a healthy body. PREVENTION is the name of the game!

Pyorrhoea

This is a disease of the gums and tooth sockets which is characterized by tender or sore gums, the formation of pus, and in some cases, loosening of the teeth.

Remedies

- Brush with goldenseal and myrrh powder.
- Rinse and gargle with tea made of goldenseal and myrrh. Put one teaspoon of each in one large glass of boiling water and steep to make tea. Also, brush gums with the tea.
- Rub the gums mornings and evenings with vitamin E oil.

Root Canal

Root Canal is the pulp-filled cavity, which also contains the nerves, in the root of a tooth. Root Canal treatment is also the procedure to replace the infected pulp in a root canal with an inert material.

The nerve in the root canal can be infected. This is often called an infected Root Canal. This may or may not cause much pain.

If the pain gets too bad or the pulp is damaged, Root Canal treatment is called for.

The treatment of the nerve in the root canal is also called Root Canal. During a root canal procedure, the nerve and pulp is removed and the inside of the tooth is cleaned and sealed.

Also see Questions 8 and 9 in the Frequently Asked Questions (Appendix A).

Teething in Infants

In order to cope with the irritation and pain that is associated with teething, rub lobelia extract, aloe vera gel, or peppermint oil on the gums.

Tooth Grinding (Bruxism)

Pent-up stress is the usual cause of tooth grinding, also known as bruxism, a common and potentially damaging process of nighttime gnashing or daytime jaw clenching. Grinding erodes tooth enamel (the protective covering of the tooth) to the point where teeth become more sensitive to hot and cold foods and drinks. It can cause severe headaches and jaw and facial pain.

Causes

- Airway obstruction, which is due to:
  o Sinusitis
  o Rhinitis
  o *Obstructive Sleep Apnea*
  o *Large tonsils and adrenals*
  o *Allergies*
- Pain (neck, shoulder, gastric and others)
- Chronic anxiety
- Side effects of certain medications
- Sometime a deficiency of calcium or vitamin B5 (pantothenic acid)

Remedies

- Herbs: chamomile and skullcap
- Sleep on your back
- Eat raw apples, celery, broccoli and carrots
- Stay away from liquor before going to bed.
- Apply a washcloth, after soaking in warm water, on your jaw. Use it as many times as you can, especially before bedtime.
- Pantothenic acid (Vitamin B5).

- Take vitamin B complex (liquid preferable) before bed for the best results.
- If nothing works, then wear a customised mouth guard while sleeping.

Teeth Grinding in Children

Some small children develop a habit of tooth grinding. You can help at bedtime by talking to them and reading a story, since it changes their focus and relaxes them. Get them involved in sports, play together with them with toys and games. Show your understanding with their challenges.

Tooth Sensitivity

Symptoms

Teeth sensitivity results from the exposure of dentin, the layer just under the enamel of the teeth.

Causes

The causes are over-brushing, incorrect brushes, small cracks in tooth, worn enamel, and receded gums.

Receded gums results in exposing microscopic tubules, little holes leading from the dentin direct to the sensitive pulp tissue at the tooth centre. It might well be that at first you don't feel any pain until the tiny tubules come into contact with air, cold, heat, sugar and these stimuli transmit signals to the pulp and... Bingo! This can create shock waves of pain. This sensation disappears as soon as the stimulus is removed, unlike the constant pounding of a toothache.

Remedies

Avoid toothpastes with whiteners since they contain harmful ingredients, which are harsh and abrasive. Read the label and use toothpaste with natural herbal ingredients and essential oils.

If you have sensitive teeth, avoid extreme hot and cold temperatures and never drink "ice-cold" drinks from the fridge. Refrain from extreme hot and cold drinks anyway as they will harm your stomach and the digestion system. Avoid hot drinks, if you have mercury fillings, as the mercury emits gas on being heated.

Try to limit acidic food, drinks and sweets since the acid can eat away at your tooth's enamel and prevent your tooth's natural healing process.

Tooth Stains

This seems to be one of the pressing problems in our society, since the oral health industry (manufacturers of toothpaste) keeps promoting white teeth that sparkle all the time "as seen on TV". Also see Tooth Whiteners, Chapter 5, Section 5.

North Americans are world champions in around the clock "brainwashing" people. People do not realize that they are paying for that "brainwashing" advertising when they are buying one of the personal care products advertised on TV, newspapers and other media.

Causes

We all start out with white, healthy, shiny teeth when we are born. Black tea and smoking are two main causes of stained teeth.

They become stained teeth by eating junk and processed food, and foods that cause stains such as berries and red wines.

However, there are situations where people develop stains even when they consume a proper diet, and in these cases, the cause is minerals in saliva.

Remedies

- Apply Baking soda on your teeth with your wet index finger and brush.

- In some cases, you probably will have to have your teeth cleaned by your dentist. If you develop stains too frequently, you may have to get your teeth cleaned every few months.

- Remember, teeth are never meant to be totally white: their natural colour is light yellow.

Toothache and Tooth Decay

Symptoms

Tooth pain triggered by eating sweets or drinking cold liquids or breathing cold air indicates the presence of decay or sensitivity due to recession of gums. This type of pain does not last long. Tooth decay rivals the common cold as a more prevalent condition and depends on three factors:

- The presence of bacteria
- The availability of sugars for the bacteria to feed on
- The vulnerability of tooth enamel

Tooth decay is not part of a normal aging or deteriorating process, as many people think; it is a bacterial disease. If heat brings on constant or short attacks of pain, chances are that the cavity has extended and reached down into the root canal. When the nerve inside the tooth becomes inflamed, tooth pain lasts longer.

Causes of Toothache

Cavities are the leading cause of toothaches. Unfortunately, cavities are exceedingly common and largely due to poor habits developed in childhood. Cavities begin when a small area of the enamel, the hard outer coating of the tooth, is demineralised from the plaque build-up. Plaque is made of bacteria that are able to penetrate the enamel. Once the enamel is eroded, the tooth pulp can be damaged which causes inflammation and toothache. If the erosion continues, the pulp is destroyed, resulting in an infected area, an abscess and ultimately, the destruction of the tooth.

Tooth sensitivity after a filling is normal for the first few days, but it should not last longer. Another cause of ache and soreness can be poking of a wisdom tooth through the gums.

Remedies for Toothache

- Boil 1 cup of chopped mulberry bark or twigs in 1-quart grape juice for ½ hour. Take 1 tablespoon, 6 times daily; keep it in your mouth for a few minutes before swallowing.
- Calendula, chamomile, peppermint and yarrow are a natural anti-inflammatory. Kava kava, St. John's Wort, white willow bark and wintergreen have analgesic properties.
- Other helpful herbal remedies are dandelion juice, elder-flower tea, sage tea, Goldenseal and Echinacea tincture.
- Soak black tea bag in hot water and keep it overnight inside the cheeks in your mouth.
- Apply (using your washed finger) a little oil of clove inserted into the cavity
- Sprinkle pepper and mustard onto a piece of cloth and rub over aching cheek.
- Mix 2 – 3 teaspoons of Himalayan crystal or sea salt in a glass of water. The salt draws out some of the fluids causing the swelling and has a general soothing effect. The salt water rinse also cleans

the area around the infected tooth and will flush out an irritating piece of rotting food which can provide immediate relief.

- Apply oil of oregano or mix it with clove and evening primrose oils. Please note that some people may not be able to tolerate oil of oregano's full strength.

Wisdom Teeth

A new study published in the "Journal of Biological Chemistry" reveals a fascinating new medical fact about wisdom teeth. Far from being a useless annoyance, wisdom teeth contain valuable tissues inside them that are capable of creating therapeutic stem cells. In the event that a person needs them, such stem cells could be used to re-grow needed tissues and organs or to treat debilitating diseases.

In 2006, some researchers first discovered that certain genes in adult cells could be reprogrammed to express themselves as fresh stem cells. Induced pluripotent stem cells (iPS), as they are called, have great therapeutic potential because they can be instructed to develop into virtually any needed adult stem cells, which can be used to promote healing.

Researchers from Japan's National Institute of Advanced Industrial Science discovered that wisdom teeth contain considerably viable "starter" cells. In addition, since most people in developed nations get their wisdom teeth removed, the process of obtaining them is simpler than it is from practically any other source.

According to a study, Hajime Ohgushi and his team gathered samples from the wisdom teeth of three donors and used them to generate iPS. In some cases, the cells proliferated 100 times more efficiently than those derived from skin, and they were capable of forming a variety of adult cell lines. Wisdom teeth can also be frozen for several years after being extracted allowing their valuable pulp to be stored for potential future use. Overall, the breakthrough research advances the cause of non-controversial iPS treatments, which show incredible promise in helping the body to heal itself.

CHAPTER 7

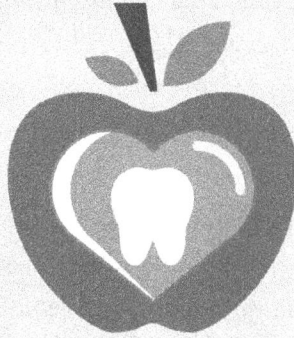

All About Mercury Fillings

A barbarous practice, the inconsistency, folly, and injury of which no words can sufficiently describe. Condemning the use of mercurial medicines.

~ A Treatise on Anatomy, Physiology, and Health (1848)

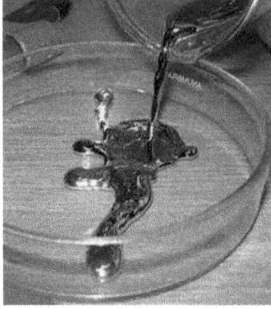

"Mercury (element) is a chemical element with symbol Hg and atomic number 80. It is commonly known as quicksilver and was formerly named hydrargyrum (/ha??dr?rd??r?m/). A heavy, silvery d-block element, mercury is the only metallic element that is liquid at standard conditions for temperature and pressure; the only other element that is liquid under these conditions is bromine, though metals such as caesium, gallium, and rubidium melt just above room temperature".

From Wikiquote.com

This chapter discusses mercury fillings as a tooth condition, systemic effects and some methods to reduce the toxicity of mercury in the body.

Section 1:
Toxicity from Mercury Fillings

Do Dental Amalgam Fillings Contain Toxic Materials?

Silver fillings (that is the name for mercury or amalgam fillings given by dentists) are made up of five different metals amalgamated together by the use of mercury that hardens into a solid mass:

- **Mercury** (accounts for 40- 50% of the complete filling)
- Silver
- Copper

- Tin
- Zinc
- Occasionally nickel

It has been shown that mercury is continuously released from mercury dental fillings in the form of mercury vapour and abraded particles.

The process is further stimulated and can be increased as much as 15 fold by:

- Chewing
- Brushing your teeth
- Drinking hot drinks
- Swishing your mouth with a chemical mouthwash or a solution of hydrogen peroxide

Many dentists believe the myth that putting poisonous mercury into the mouths of patients is perfectly safe. Fortunately, there are many dentists that agree that all of the elements comprising dental amalgam are toxic. Mercury has the ability to pass rapidly into the body into the blood and into the body cells and remain there!

> Mercury is extremely poisonous. Published research from two scientists at Utah State University concluded that mercury is more toxic than lead, cadmium and even arsenic, accumulating over time in the various tissues of the body, especially the brain and kidneys. In human autopsy studies, it has been found that there is a direct correlation between the amount of mercury found in the brain and the number of mercury amalgam fillings in the teeth. Mercury is one of the most toxic substances known to man.

What are the systemic effects in the body?

- Neurological: frequent or chronic headaches.
- Fine tremors (hands, feet, lips, eyelids and tongue).

- Immunological: allergies, rhinitis (inflammation of the nose), sinusitis, asthma, lymphadenopathy, especially cervical or neck.

- Endocrine: subnormal temperatures, cold, clammy skin, especially hands and feet, excessive perspiration.

- Other: muscle weakness, chronic fatigue, hypoxia (lack of oxygen), anorexia, joint pains, anaemia, edema (swelling), loss of weight, in severe cases - hallucinations and manic depression.

Besides mercury amalgam fillings, we absorb mercury from the following sources:

- Mercury derived from air
- Water
- Fish, such as tuna
- Clothes and paints

Dr. Murray J. Vimy, DMD, Clinical Associate Professor, Faculty of Medicine, University of Calgary is one of the foremost mercury toxicity researchers and author of the book titled: *Your Toxic Teeth: A guide to Mercury Poisoning from Dental Fillings.* Here, is an excerpt from his book:

"The scientific facts reviewed in this book are compelling. There is little scientific debate about the validity of these facts within the medical research community. However, the American and Canadian Dental Associations and their corporate dental manufacturing partners, under the direction of the bureaucrats and dental academics, are waging a media war to sway public opinion. Opposition from organised dentistry to the revelation has been swift. Claims by self-appointed dental "experts" that mercury/silver fillings are safe flies in the face of a growing body of experimental medical research evidence published in respected peer-adjudicated medical research journals."

Furthermore, there are other pioneer dentists, who have discovered over three decades ago the toxic dangers of mercury amalgam fillings, such as Dr. Hal A. Huggins and Dr. Tom McGuire. Books by these and other authors are listed in Appendix E.

Please also read the article in Natural Life Magazine, January/February 1997 issue with the title: *Mercury Fillings: A Time Bomb in Your Head* by

Charles W. Moore, naturallifemagazine.com/9702/mercury.htm

> Countries like Denmark, Norway, New Zealand, and Sweden have banned mercury amalgam-fillings. Austria, Canada and Germany have issued restriction on using them. There is a growing movement, based on many scientific studies, that other countries will follow in the future either to restrict the use or to ban them. However, the mercury manufacturers have strong lobbies approaching governments; therefore, it will take a while before more countries start further actions.

In the US, leading dentists have formed holistic dental associations (see Appendix) that promote alternative fillings to mercury amalgam fillings and here in Canada there is a trend of holistic dentists doing the same.

Some forward thinking dentists are spearheading a movement to ban mercury fillings in North America. Ironically, both the FDA (Food & Drug Administration, USA) and Health Canada consider mercury amalgams safe.

The International Academy of Oral Medicine & Toxicology offers a shocking video called "Smoking Teeth" that clearly shows mercury vapour off gassing from mercury fillings, even with minimal stimulation like chewing or tooth brushing. How much mercury? One thousand times the EPA's (Environmental Protection Association) maximum allowable mercury limit for air. The video is a must-see! www.youtube. com/watch?v=9ylnQ-T7oiA

Also search for David Kennedy, DDS on http://www.youtube.com

To learn more about mercury amalgam fillings please check the following websites:

International Academy of Oral Medicine and Toxicology to see over 50 videos and many articles, etc. www.iaomt.org/

Dr. Tom McGuire www.mercuryfreenow.com/tom/tomart.html

Dental Wellness Institute www.dentalwellness4u.com

The Mercury Papers - The Most Expensive Medical Mistake in the History of the World

www.positivehealth.com/issue/issue-178-january-2011 **www. wholisticresearch.com/info/artshow.php3?artid=20**

In the interest of informed consent, please pursue the following links, which present opposing viewpoints on the issue of mercury fillings:

Policy Statement of the Royal College of Dental Surgeons of Ontario bit.ly/RCDSOHg

Appendix B lists many Holistic Dental Organizations. Some websites dealing with Dental Mercury Dangers are listed in Appendix C.

Section 2:
How to Reduce the Toxic Load
of Amalgam Fillings

There are many ways to detox the body, such as food, herbs, supplements, drugs and sweat therapy.

Similarly herbs, sweat therapy and chelation therapy are some of the ways used to reduce the toxic load from mercury.

Chlorella

Chlorella is a type of algae that grows in fresh water. The whole plant is used to make nutritional supplements and medicine. Mercury is preferentially attracted to the cell wall of the unicellular organism chlorella.

Garlic & MSM

Mercury can bind to sulfhydryl groups in **garlic** or sulphur in the form of MSM (methyl sulfonyl methane).

Milk Thistle

Milk thistle or a milk thistle combination that cleanses the liver, purifies the blood, detoxifies the liver and kidneys and boosts the immune system also reduces the toxicity of mercury.

Sweat Therapy

Far-infrared sauna treatment for whole body detoxification is recommended.

Chelation Therapy

The clinical goal is to convert the mercury into a state that enables it to be removed from the cells and eliminated from the brain, connective tissues, lymph system, liver, kidneys and gastrointestinal tract.

EDTA Therapy

EDTA (ethylene diamine tetraacetic acid, edetate sodium) which has been available in Canada now for several years and has been used to help remove various heavy metals from the body. However, EDTA therapy is not without controversy.

www.cancer.org/Treatment/TreatmentsandSideEffects/
ComplementaryandAlternativeMedicine/
PharmacologicalandBiologicalTreatment/chelation-therapy

Cilantro (Coriander)

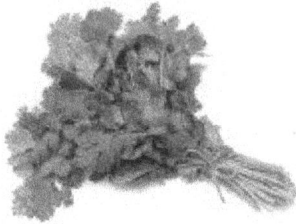

Since Roman times cilantro/coriander (Coriandrumm sativum) has been used as food and medicine. It acts as a reducing agent changing the charge on the intracellular mercury to a neutral state, allowing the mercury to diffuse its concentration gradient into the connective tissue. Some experts believe the use of cilantro dates back to 5000 BC. References to cilantro can be found in the Sanskrit writings, and the seeds were often placed in Egyptian tombs.

www.health-inspiration.com/html/cilantro.html

A study by Dr. Yoshiaki Omura from the Heart Disease Research Foundation, New York, N.Y. has discovered that the cilantro herb will detoxify mercury from neural tissue. This is a remarkable discovery!

Today, cilantro is cultivated in tropical and subtropical countries throughout the world including North & South America, Europe and the Mediterranean area. Besides detoxifying metals (especially mercury) cilantro has other properties and uses: antispasmodic, appetizer, aromatic, carminative and stomachic. It can also be applied externally for rheumatism and painful joints.

Cilantro Blend

Cilantro blend contains yellow dock and cilantro.

Yellow dock (Rumex crispus) has been known as a medicinal plant since ancient times and was used as a laxative or a mild astringent tonic. American Indians applied crushed yellow dock leaves to boil and the pulverized roots to cuts. In the nineteenth century, yellow dock was considered a "blood purifier" and was prescribed for eruptive diseases, such as scrofula and skin problems. The cilantro blend works through increasing the ability of the liver and related organs to strain and purify the blood and lymph system. It achieves its tonic properties through an astringent purification of the blood supply to the glands and acts as a cleansing herb for the lymphatic system.

Cilantro blend contains yellow dock to help drain the mercury from the connective tissue. The blend also significantly increases our ability to clear up recurring infections, both viral and bacterial. Bioactive cilantro blend (coriander/yellow dock) herbal tincture is an inexpensive, easy way to remove or chelate toxic metals from the nervous system and body tissues.

> According to the American Academy of Environmental Medicine the average person has 287 toxins in their body. It might interest you: In a blood analysis of a former Canadian Federal Health Minister Toni Clement they found fifty-five chemicals in his body.

Dr. Omura performed another study in which three amalgam fillings were removed from a patient using all of the precautions available to prevent absorption of mercury from the amalgam removal. Even with strong air and water suctioning, water rinses and a rubber dental dam, significant amounts of mercury were later found in the patient's lungs, kidneys, endocrine organs, liver and heart.

No mercury was detected in these areas prior to the date of removal. It is, therefore, necessary to continue using the herbal tinctures after the removal of mercury amalgam fillings, and the far-infrared sauna to further detoxify your body.

Section 3:
Removing Mercury Fillings

Protection of the patient from additional exposure to mercury is of the utmost concern during the removal of mercury fillings. This is especially true of the mercury toxic patient. The goal of this protocol is to minimize for the patient, practitioner and environment any additional exposure to mercury.

Mercury vapour not only is absorbed by the lungs through inhalation, but also through intact skin.

Review the international safety card on mercury:

www.cdc.gov/niosh/ipcsneng/neng0056.html

Protocols for Removing Mercury Fillings

The protocols given below, turned into questionnaires are recommended by the **IAOMT (International Academy of Oral Medicine and Toxicology).**

When you are considering the removal of mercury fillings, ask if the dentist is properly trained in Mercury Removal Procedures. Responsible dentists belong to some professional organizations supporting such procedures though they may not practice all of the protocols.

The questions are in four categories:

A. Dealing with Patient

B. Compatibility of Replacement Material

C. Dealing with the Treatment Environment

D. Dealing with the Follow-up

A. Dealing with the Patient

1. Before the procedure: Do you provide or recommend the patient to take anything before, during or after the procedure, such as IV Vitamin C, nutritional supplements or detox methods.

2. Do you use pre and post-oral rinse with a mercury binding agent (e.g. Oral Detox Pro or Chlorella)?

3. How do you prevent mercury residue from entering the mouth?

4. Do you use a rubber dam? What type?

   The rubber dam, particularly made of nitrile, catches most of the pieces of old filling and dust created by the drilling. It also helps to prevent the soft tissues of the mouth from absorbing mercury vapour.

5. Do you promote chewing on Chlorella or place liquid Chlorella in mouth and isolate the area being worked on with a cotton roll or gauze.

6. Take activated charcoal capsules to absorb toxins and other chemicals in the body.

7. Do you use a face cloth over the eyes or full safety glasses and full body protective coverings?

8. Do you provide the patient with an alternate air supply delivered nasally?

9. How do you drill out the amalgam? Do you section and remove amalgam in large chunks? (The use of thin sharp burs to "chunk out" the filling will minimize the amount of amalgam drilled).

10. Do you use high volume water cooling during use of air rotor?

11. Do you use a high volume suction to remove particles, air, water and mercury vapour from the mouth.

12. Do you use "Clean Up" by Bio Probe?

B. Compatibility of Replacement Material

1. Do you do serum or other Biocompatibility testing to determine if the recommended replacement material will be compatible?

2. Do you have further training in the mercury fillings removal and/or dental clearance?

C. Dealing with the Treatment Environment

1. Do you use full protective draping for the patient?

2. Is the water in your dental practice filtered, de-mineralized and de-ionized?

3. Do you use a mercury vapour ionizing system?

4. Do you use a high-powered dental suction system?

5. Do you and your assistant wear mercury-protective clothing that is properly disposed of following amalgam removal? Do you use Nitrile gloves to protect you?

6. Do you use a respirator or a separate air supply to protect you?

D. Dealing with the Follow-up

1. Do you refer for acupressure to rebalance energetics and lymphatic massage after treatment?

2. Do you recommend follow-up chelation and detoxification protocol?

3. Do you recommend holistic health practitioners or a functional MD?

7. Do you provide nutritional counselling to support the immune system and enhance the body's detoxification ability before the removal and after the removal?

A dentist may not practice all protocols mentioned which is acceptable as long as you are protected from the exposure of mercury.

Summary of Protocols for Removing Mercury Fillings

This is based on recommendations of the International Academy of Oral Medicine and Toxicology (IAOMT), Dr. Hal Huggins, and other prominent holistic dental organizations. Some dentists have their own and may include some or all of the steps mentioned below:

1 **Rubber Dam** - This is a thin sheet of rubber that isolates the tooth/ teeth being worked on and helps prevent particles and bacteria from entering the soft tissue of the mouth.

2   **Negative Ion Generators** - When removing amalgam fillings, the vapor from the fillings releases into the air. The negative ion generators help to capture the mercury in a filter thus reducing exposure to patient, dentist, and assistant.

3.   **Sequential Removal of Fillings** - Measuring the electrical current using a Rita Meter and removing the most negative current fillings first, allowing a set of 4 healing endocrine glands to be stimulated therefore promoting healing.

4.   **Immune Compatible Filling Materials** - A serum compatibility test of your blood to be tested against most dental materials in use today. Only those materials that report minimal challenge to your immune system will be selected.

5.   **Oxygen for the Patient to Breathe** - To greater eliminate the possibility of breathing in mercury vapor.

6.   **IV Vitamin C** - Provided for protection against fumes and vapors that can be absorbed or inhaled as fillings are removed. IV Vitamin C is especially necessary during oral surgery. Bacteria and toxins release into your blood stream during oral surgery and the vitamin C can aid in neutralizing their damaging properties.

7.   **Conscious Sedation** - This is an intravenous procedure that puts you in the twilight zone. This allows all work to be able to be completed in one appointment to the delight of your immune system.

8.   **Massage** - Generally applied a day or two before revision. The purpose is to stimulate the release of ionic calcium needed for healing after surgery. Massage also helps to stimulate your white blood cells, which are needed after a dental revision.

9.   **Acupressure** - Immediately after dental revision, acupressure has the ability of reintroducing your nervous system to your muscular system. The normal impulses that connect these parts of your anatomy get "scrambled" during dental procedures. This procedure has also shown to alleviate pain therefore very little pain medication may be necessary.

Review videos demonstrating the Mercury Removal Procedure at IAOMT:

iaomt.org/basics/

See Appendix for Additional websites regarding **Dental Mercury Dangers.**

Section 4:
Top Ten Reasons to Support Mercury-Free Dentistry

1. Amalgam pollutes our environment

- **WATER**: via water from dental clinic releases and human waste. Some jurisdictions such as Ontario now mandate that all dental offices MUST have a mercury separator most of which prevent 99% of mercury from making it into the sewage (if used properly).

- **AIR**: via cremation, dental clinic emissions, sludge incineration, and respiration; and

- **LAND:** via landfills, burials, and fertilizer. Once in the environment, dental mercury is converted to its even more toxic form: methyl mercury and becomes a major source of mercury in the fish people eat. Dental mercury in the environment can cause brain damage and neurological problems, especially for children and the unborn babies, according to the United States Environmental Protection Agency.

2. Amalgam endangers our health

Amalgam emits mercury vapour even after it is implanted into the body. This mercury is bio-accumulative, and it crosses the placenta to accumulate in fetuses as well. Dental amalgam's mercury is a known health risk, especially for children, fetuses, nursing infants, and especially for people with impaired kidney function. Even the U.S. Food and Drug Administration concedes that the developing neurological systems of children and fetuses are more susceptible to 'the neurotoxic effects of mercury vapour' - and that there is no evidence that amalgam is safe for these populations.

3. Amalgam endangers dental workers

Due to mercury exposure from amalgam in the workplace; studies have shown that dental workers have elevated systemic mercury levels. Few of these dental workers – mostly women of childbearing age - are given protective garb or air masks to minimize their exposure to mercury; many are not aware of the risks of occupational mercury exposure. As a result, dental workers have reported neurological problems, reproductive failures, and birth defects caused by amalgam in the workplace.

4. Amalgam damages teeth

Placing amalgam require the removal of a significant amount of healthy tooth matter. This removal, in turn, weakens the overall tooth structure which increases the need for future dental work. On top of that, amalgam fillings - which expand and contract over time - crack teeth and once again create the need for still more dental work.

5. Amalgam is frequently implanted without informed consent

Most dentists do not inform consumers that amalgam contains mercury. As a result, over 76% of consumers do not know that amalgam is mainly mercury according to Zogby polls. But once they are informed, 77% of people do not want mercury fillings - and they were even willing to pay more to avoid this unnecessary source of mercury exposure.

6. Amalgam perpetuates social injustice

While middle class consumers opt for mercury-free filling materials; people in developing nations, low-income families, minorities, military personnel, prisoners, and people with disabilities are still subjected to amalgam. Racial minorities are more likely to receive amalgam; for example, dentists place almost 25% more mercury fillings in American Indian patients than in white patients. In his testimony before Congress, former Virginia State NAACP president Emmitt Carlton described this injustice as "choice for the rich, mercury for the poor."

7. Amalgam costs taxpayers

Taxpayers foot the bill for the environmental clean-up of amalgam and the medical care associated with mercury-related health problems. In some jurisdictions, with no regulations to separate mercury, the dentists who dump their mercury into our environment and our bodies are not held financially responsible.

8. Amalgam is diverted to illegal gold mining

Amalgam is commonly shipped to developing countries labelled for dental use, but then it is diverted to illegal use in artisanal and small-scale gold mining. Not only are the miners exposed to the risks of mercury poisoning, but the dental mercury they use to extract gold is released into the environment.

9. Amalgam is interchangeable with mercury-free filling materials.

Amalgam is interchangeable with numerous other filling materials – including resin composites, compomers, and glass ionomers - that have rendered amalgam completely unnecessary for any clinical situation. In fact, the mercury-free alternatives have made amalgam so non-essential that entire nations, such as the Scandinavian countries, have banned the use of amalgam. Developing nations have benefitted from modern mercury-free techniques, such as atraumatic restorative treatment (ART), which only cost half as much as amalgam and make dental care more accessible.

10. Amalgam drives up the price of mercury-free alternatives

The continued use of amalgam keeps the price of mercury-free filling materials high by decreasing demand for these alternatives. As use of mercury-free materials increases, their price is expected to decrease even further.

Source "*Campaign for Mercury-Free Dentistry*" www.toxicteeth.org/

CHAPTER 8

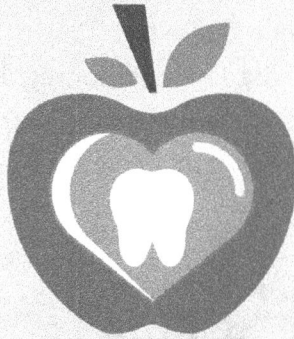

Understanding
Dental Practice

If suffering brought wisdom,
the dentist's office would be full of luminous ideas.
~Mason Cooley

Now is the time to delve into the practice of dentistry.

In this Chapter will explore and contrast conventional dental practice with the holistic/biologic dentistry. This is followed by "How an Holistic dentist will examine a patient thoroughly to assess any systemic oral link". We will also look at some dental restoration procedures and the material used. Finally a word about various dental specialists and their role.

Section 1:
Understanding Holistic
Dental Practice

We believe that the conventional allopathic approach to medicine has fallen short of the aspect of the total integrative health of a patient; therefore consider bringing alternative therapies and integrative medicine to any health practice.

This section will provide you with some understanding of a holistic hygienist and a holistic dental practice and how do they differ from mainstream practice. Biological dentist and mercury-free dentist are terms also used for holistic dentists. Similarly, some holistic hygienists also use the term Systemic hygienist or Integrative hygienist.

The objective is to provide you with some criteria to consider when you are shopping for a new dentist or a hygienist or comparing the services of your existing dental care professional.

A holistic hygienist or dentist thinks about healing the whole body via the mouth versus just treating the mouth. This mouth and body connection is also called the Oral Systemic Link.

> "No informed dentist will deny the connection between oral health and total health, particularly when it comes to heart diseases, diabetes, etc. But traditional dentists do little, in our opinion, about this issue."
> Dr. Oksana Sawiak

Holistic dentistry (including dental hygiene) is an approach to dental treatment that primarily cares for the patient's health and safety from both a conventional, as well as, an alternative healthcare point of view. The mouth is the gateway to the stomach and a mirror of what is happening inside the body.

Section 2:
Distinction from Conventional Practice

> The difference is philosophical, as well as in treatment. Holistic dentistry relates to removing major obstacles to healthy living and accelerates recovery from chronic illness. It stresses the relationship of oral health to total wellness because of the interconnection of the teeth to the organs of the body, not just looking at 'symptoms' for answers.

Some of the distinctions are given below:

1. Holistic dentists prefer the overview of a panoramic x-ray to a full-mouth series of x-rays. This lets the dentist see impacted teeth, root fragments, bits of mercury buried in the bone and deep infections. A full mouth series is more likely to miss them. On the other hand, individual bitewing or periapical x-rays have a higher

resolution and can thus render more detail. The total radiation dose from a panoramic x-ray is much less than from a full-mouth series.

2. Placing crowns on teeth to protect or strengthen them is not always recommended. Certainly artificial crowns strengthen damaged teeth against breakage, but they require more removal of tooth structure than does a large filling. There is a trade-off here, which the holistic dentist is more likely to take into account.

3. No dental amalgam or mercury fillings. Instead, a holistic dentist will use non-metallic alternative replacements, such as porcelain, composite or Zirconium.

4. Root Canal Therapy is typically not recommended by a holistic dentist, and if they do, it is performed after the canal is fully sterilized. Some holistic dentists are using Ozone Treatment Therapy for thorough sterilization. Additionally, a root filling that does not shrink away from the walls of the canal is used.

5. Fluoride is not recommended.

6. Dental materials for fillings and other procedures are (often) tested for biocompatibility with the person's body.

7. Holistic dentists recognize the existence of cavitations (holes, cavities) left in the jaw bone by extracted teeth, root canal infections, etc. They try to prevent cavitations when extracting a tooth by removing the periodontal ligament that fastens the tooth to the bone. Conventional dentistry for some reason ignores cavitations.

8. Advice on nutritional supplements and detoxification of residual mercury deposits in body tissues, prior to, during and after amalgam removal.

9. Advice and treatment from other holistic practitioners (such as holistic nutritionists, holistic oral surgeons, chiropractors, and osteopaths) is sought and considered as an integral part of the dental practice.

10. Holistic dentists believe in detoxification of the body, as well as dental revision.

The next Section consists of the following:

- Patient Examination
- Protocols to Remove Mercury Fillings
- Metal-Free Replacement Alternatives
- Dental Professional Organizations

Section 3:
Patient Examination
by a Holistic Dentist

The holistic dental practitioner will take the time to review the medical and dental health history, gather information about the Oral Systemic Link (see Glossary). A holistic hygienist or dentist will consider what the root causes are and why the teeth are decaying, why the gum tissues are bleeding or why the oral tissues are inflamed.

There are two types of examination/assessments:

- Outside the mouth called Extra-Oral Examination
- Inside the mouth called Intra-Oral Examination

Extra-Oral Examination

- Observes imbalance in posture, face and head. Check the neck for swollen glands, tension and tenderness in muscles, skin colouring, nerve paralysis, lymphatic drainage, opening of the jaw, signs of abnormalities that need to be noted.
- Review medical history and blood pressure.

Intra-Oral Examination

The focus of the Intra-Oral Examination is on the hard and soft tissues. This can also be done by a hygienist. They check soft tissue (gums and tongue) and hard tissue (teeth, bone underneath the soft tissue, upper jaw palate).

- Check for swelling, bleeding upon touch, signs of redness, plaque coating on teeth, tartar build-up locations on the teeth, cavities in the teeth.

- Check for suspected cancerous tissue on the jaws, palate and all soft tissues like the tongue, inside the cheeks, back of the throat and the uvula.

- Check the tongue for coating, colour, size, anatomical patterns, and teeth marks. Look underneath the tongue for swelling, blood circulation.

- Check teeth for wear patterns, colour, filling condition and history, crown margins at the gum line (if there is any irritation).

- Assess the type of material used in the restorative work and its impact on general health.

- Some practitioners also use the Tooth and Organ Chart to assess the connection of teeth with patients' health conditions.

Equipment Used for Examination

There are two groups of equipment:

1. Clinical hygiene equipment (Used for cleaning the teeth).

2. Test and diagnostic equipment (Used for screening for mouth and body inflammation connections). The equipment will include:

- Microscope.

- A computer software or process such as the Oral Systemic Links (see glossary).

- Digital low-dose x-ray equipment including panoramic.

- Intra oral camera.

- Infrared thermal imaging camera for head and neck area (Thermography).

- pH measurement like litmus paper.

- Strep Mutans test.

Section 4:
Types of Tooth Restorations

There are three basic restorations:

- Inlays and Onlays (Indirect fillings)
- Direct filling
- Dental Crown

Inlays and Onlays (Indirect fillings)

Inlays and Onlays are indirect dental restorations that reinforce an existing tooth (mostly chewing surface) that is too damaged to support a filling, but not damaged enough to require a crown.

Traditional fillings are made directly in the mouth, while inlays and onlays are made in a dental lab or milled by machine. Inlays and onlays are both made from a mould so they fit your tooth perfectly. Inlays fit tightly within the prepared cavity, so they are smaller than dental crowns and onlays.

Onlays are slightly larger – larger than regular fillings – and they cover the whole chewing area and overlap the edge of the teeth so that they protect the cusps of the tooth. Onlays are similar to crowns and cover more of the tooth making them more extensive in coverage than inlays, but less so than crowns.

Dental crowns

Dental crowns, also known as caps, preserve the functionality of damaged teeth. A dental crown may be used to protect a cracked tooth, restore functionality of a tooth with excessive decay or replace a pre-existing crown. The purpose of a dental crown is to encase a needy tooth with a custom-designed material.

Dental crowns and fillings are made of the following material:

- Precious Metal (Gold)

- Mixed Alloys (palladium and nickel mixed with gold and non-precious metals
- Silver Amalgam: mercury mixed with silver, tin, zinc
- Metal-Free (plastic, resin, composite and porcelain)

Metal-Free Replacement Alternatives

The following non-metallic materials are used for tooth restorations:

- Porcelain
- Composite
- Ceramic
- Zirconia

Porcelain

Tooth restorations made from porcelain are stronger than traditional fillings because they are cemented or bonded to your tooth rather than packed into a cavity. Reinforced all-porcelain crowns have now been available for over ten years. They are not to be confused with porcelain bonded metal crowns which are more common, but which often have nickel and palladium as one of the metals used within the alloy. Many people believe they have porcelain crowns when in reality there is a metal core underneath the porcelain. If there is a marrow band of silver at the gum margin on the inside of the crown, then there is metal under the porcelain. Porcelain fillings are often called inlays, ceramic or Cerec restorations.

Composite

A composite is made of a very hard 'plastic'. Most of the plastics contain BPA (a toxic substance), but the amounts are negligible and all "free BPA" is removed when the filling is polished.

Ceramic

A ceramic restoration has real advantages if someone is allergic or sensitive to petrochemicals. However, they are very hard and may cause abrasion of the opposing teeth.

Zirconia

These are a non-conductive oxide of zirconium, fashioned by computer, which replaces the metal or gold part of the older type of crown, inlays or onlays. Porcelain is still bonded to the Zirconia to provide the correct shape and aesthetics. Zirconia is 100% biocompatible. It is inert, and the body does not reject Zirconia so you do not have to worry about allergies or adverse reactions. Zirconia crowns and implants are rapidly becoming a new choice for many dentists. Zirconia is hard like a diamond, resistant to corrosion and similar in strength to steel.

When selecting a replacement for restoration, explore with your dentist, the pros and cons of each option, such as elasticity, shear strength, compressive strength, and susceptibility to load failure. It is also necessary to consider the location of the restoration in the mouth (e.g. front tooth, molar). In some situations porcelain crowns may break in the back teeth.

Replacement alternatives may contain BPA, read: www.rodale.com/bpa-fillings

Section 5:
A Word About Dental Specialists

General Dentist

A general dentist is your primary care dental provider. This dentist diagnoses, treats, and manages your overall oral health care needs, including gum care, root canals, fillings, crowns, veneers, bridges, and preventive education.

Dental Anesthesiologist

A Dental Anesthesiologist is a dentist who has specialized in the practice of Anesthesiology for dental treatments. Anaesthesiology is the branch of dentistry (and medicine) involving the use of medications and other agents that create a reversible lack of awareness, blocking of pain and relieving of anxiety and stress for patients receiving dental treatments.

Endodontist

Endodontics is the branch of dentistry that is concerned with what goes on inside your tooth. In fact the word is derived from the Greek word for inside (endo) and tooth (odons). Inside your hard tooth is a space that is filled with soft tissue. This tissue contains blood vessels, nerves and various types of cells that played an important role in the development of the tooth.

Oral and Maxillofacial Surgeon

Oral and Maxillofacial Surgeons are involved in the diagnosis, surgical and non-surgical treatment of disorders, diseases, injuries and defects, involving the functional and aesthetic aspects of the hard and soft tissues of the oral and maxillofacial regions and related structures (entire face, mouth, and jaw area). They also treat patients with tumours and cysts of the jaws.

Orthodontics and Dentofacial Orthopedics

The Specialty of Orthodontics and Dentofacial Orthopedics is the branch of dentistry that specializes in the diagnosis, prevention and treatment of dental and facial irregularities. The technical term for these problems is "malocclusion". The practice of orthodontics uses corrective appliances (retainers and/or braces) to bring teeth, lips and jaws into proper alignment and achieve facial balance

"Malocclusion" encompasses crooked, crowded or protruding teeth which do not fit together properly. Literally, the word means "bad bite".

Most malocclusions are inherited. These include crowding of teeth, too much space between teeth, extra or missing teeth, cleft palate and a variety of irregularities of the jaws and face.

Pediatrics Dentist

Pediatric dentists are dental specialists who provide routine, primary and comprehensive dental care for infants, children, adolescents and special needs patients. The pediatric dentist offers children an early and positive start for a lifetime of good dental health. The child's first dental visit should occur by their first birthday.

Pediatric dentists are considered the "pediatricians" of dentistry. Dental decay is the most common chronic disease in children and without proper care, can affect a child's overall general health.

Periodontist

Periodontics is the branch of dentistry concerned with the diagnosis, prevention and treatment of the diseases and conditions of the supporting and surrounding tissues of the teeth or their substitutes. The term is derived from the Greek word peri, for around, and odont, for tooth.

Prosthodontist

Prosthodontics is concerned with the diagnosis, restoration and maintenance of oral function, comfort, appearance and health of the patient by the restoration of the natural teeth and/or the replacement of missing teeth and contiguous oral and maxillofacial tissues with artificial substitutes.

Adapted from, Ontario Dental Association

www.oda.on.ca/you-your-dentist/specialties92

CHAPTER 9

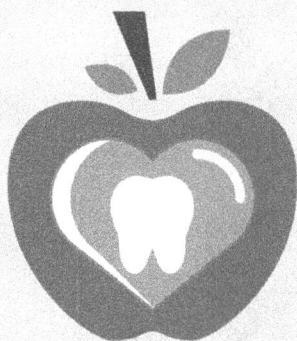

Assessing Your Oral Health

"Health is a state of complete physical, mental and social
well-being and not merely the absence of disease or infirmity".
~World Health Organization, 1948

We have provided knowledge and guidance to have a healthy mouth and body, now it is time for you to create a road map to achieve it. Just like any journey, you want to assess your conditions before you start your journey, so we are devoting this chapter for you to assess your oral health and also help you choose dental health practitioners who can help you achieve your health goals.

The aim is to make you aware of excellent oral health.

Section 1:
Assess Your Oral Health

Before paying for a dental check-up, you can identify, on your own, the issues that need to be addressed for complete dental and general health.

This assessment will give you a strong indication of your current oral and dental health conditions.

Each assessment is marked by:

☑ to indicate 'Good Oral Health' or

☒ to indicate 'Poor Oral Health'.

Give yourself +1 for each ☑ applicable to you and -1 for each ☒ applicable to you.

There are two ways to use these assessments:

1. Sum up all +1s and all -1s and see if you have a positive or negative score. The positive score indicates better oral health; the larger the number the better the health.

2. Simply use the assessments to make you aware of the factors involved in achieving or maintaining optimal dental health.

This assessment consists of 123 points grouped into 19 numbered questionnaires or areas. There are five categories of questionnaires.

- Part A: Self-Examination of Your Mouth
- Part B: Procedures Done on Your Teeth
- Part C: Symptoms of Your Mercury Fillings Toxicity
- Part D: Routines and Lifestyle Issues
- Part E: Self-Examination Procedures for Oral Cancer

You may find this section much more informative than what you will get from a dental practitioner, but still it does not replace his/her expert observation. You may take your concerns, gained from this assessment, to your practitioner to get his/her expert opinion.

DISCLAIMER

Presence of any symptom or condition is subjective and non-professional. The aim of self-assessment is to make you aware of the factors involved, but not to alarm you. You are strongly advised to take your assessment and any concerns to your dental and healthcare professionals.

Part A: Self-Examination of Your Mouth

1. Look in a mirror before you even open your mouth:
    ☒ Do your lips close over your teeth or do you need to strain to keep your mouth closed?

This mouth breathing condition can be caused by the following factors:

- Allergies
- Sinus problems
- Polyps
- Neck and spinal problems
- An extremely short upper lip
- Effects of a thumb sucking habit

- Sleep apnea
- Discrepancies between tooth-size and jaw-size; an orthodontic issue

All of the above can cause us to breathe through the mouth therefore making lips, gum tissues and teeth dry. They should be moist at all times. Dried out gums and teeth become more prone to infections and encourage an increase of plaque and decalcification of teeth.

2. Do you see:

   ☒ Cracks or areas of redness in the corners of the mouth that do not heal?

Research from Rice University shows that 70% of all people are affected by Candida, a systemic fungal infection. It is often found in colonies in the intestines, mouths or on the skin. Overgrowth of yeast, known as Candida, can be due to the overuse of antibiotics, our preference for a highly processed diet and prolific intake of sweets and stress. Candida is a nasty fungus that is hard to get rid of and can persist in causing cracks in the corners of mouth, called angular cheilitis, or to create a cushion of red inflamed sore tissue under a denture. Candida can also be due to deficiency of certain nutrients, such as iron, zinc and vitamin B2. A low level of Candida is normal and not harmful.

3. Now look into your mouth and check if you have:

   ☒ Red gums
   ☒ Bleeding gums
   ☒ Swollen or irritated gums
   ☒ Receding gums with roots exposed (teeth looking longer)

These conditions are caused by the following:

- Gum infection with bacteria, fungus or parasites.
- Poor oral hygiene (the earliest transfer of bacteria, Strep mutans, is from mother to the baby by kissing on the lips or licking the soother or bottle nipple).

- Sharing saliva from an infected partner or family member through utensils, foods and drinks and kissing.

4. Your Teeth and Mouth Conditions

Do you suffer from any of the following conditions?

☒ Bad breath (you have to ask someone to tell you) or bad taste in your mouth: Mostly caused by gum infections and cavities.

☒ Cavities: Caused by bacteria, fungus, sweets and poor oral hygiene.

☒ Exposed roots of teeth: Caused by fungus and bruxism (tooth grinding and/or clenching).

☒ Grinding or clenching teeth: Caused by stress, parasites, imbalance in the neck or spine, or a high spot in a restoration and airway issues.

☒ Headaches, earaches, neck pain, and jaw joint pain (clicking/cracking): Are often caused by bad jaw to jaw relationship, TMJD (Temporomandibular Joint Disorder), especially after trauma like whiplash or sports injuries. Hidden jaw infections (cavitations) can be a cause for unexplained headache and migraine.

☒ Loose, tipped or shifting teeth: Caused by gum infection eating away the bone which supports the teeth.

☒ Loss of enamel: You can wear enamel off by grinding your teeth or chewing extremely fibrous and rough foods (like aboriginal or raw diets). Acids which are held against teeth like 'sucking on lemons' will decalcify enamel. Aggressive scaling with metal instruments can wear enamel away.

A tooth interference problem can cause loss of gum and bone support. If a tooth is rocked by another tooth hitting it before the mouth fully closes down (like in chewing) the enamel around the gum line will break down in a wedge like shape. Many dentists and hygienists mistake these 'abfraction lesions' for toothbrush abrasion.

The greatest damage to enamel is caused by too much ingested fluoride (fluorosis). The teeth will form with spots that look opaque white or even brown. Dental fluorosis is becoming more and more prevalent due to wide use of fluoridation of water and inclusion of fluoride in many oral health products.

☒ Tooth Sensitivity to hot, cold and/or sweet: Teeth become sensitive when roots get exposed because the gums have receded due to infection, surgery or a traumatic bite. Another common cause is a reaction to the chemicals in commercial whitening toothpastes.

If the tooth is sensitive to cold or sweets, it often indicates a cavity. A cracked tooth on the other hand will be sensitive to biting and cold.

A tooth that hurts to bite or gets worse with hot, but relieved by cold is abscessed. Take care of it right away by seeing a dentist if you want to avoid severe consequences to your health.

☒ Teeth or fillings breaking: Chewing ice cracks enamel. Using your teeth as a tool, instead of using scissors or a bottle opener or a nail file, will chip or break your teeth. Buck teeth of a thumb sucker or mouth breather are more prone to trauma and breakage.

Another possible reason for tooth breakage is amalgam fillings because amalgam fillings expand with heat and contract with cold. Since amalgam fillings contain 50% mercury, they expand with hot soup or drinks and contract with very cold foods. Heavily filled teeth are not pliable so they crack. Eventually a whole ¼ or ½ could break away.

☒ Yellow or grey coloured teeth: Grey bands in teeth are a consequence of tetracycline (antibiotics) used during the time when teeth were developing in their buds. These tetracycline stains cannot be bleached out successfully.

Yellow teeth may be genetic or from too much iron from the water. Smoking, wine and infections will also cause teeth to go yellow or brown, but these stains are removable.

As we age, our enamel gets thinner and our dentin denser thus our teeth get darker yellow or brownish.

Part B: Dental Procedures Done on Your Teeth

5.   Restorative and Corrective Procedures:

Take stock of all work done on your teeth (dig up your dental history files). Any procedure done is an indication of previously poor oral health. Below are some examples of such procedures:

- ☒ Any Oral Surgery
- ☒ Bone Grafting
- ☒ Crowns/Caps
- ☒ Dental Bonding for Cosmetics
- ☒ Dentures (Prosthetics)
- ☒ Endodontic (Root Canal) Therapy
- ☒ Extractions
- ☒ Implants
- ☒ Inlays or Onlays
- ☒ Laser Treatments
- ☒ Mercury Fillings or Any Other Fillings
- ☒ Orthognathic (Jaw Repositioning) Surgery
- ☒ Periodontal (Gum) Surgery
- ☒ Temporomandibular Joint Disorder (TMJD)
- ☒ Tooth Whitening

6.   Preventive Procedures

These are preventive procedures, so any of the following procedures indicates 'positive' results:

- ☑ **Curettage** (cleaning the diseased soft disease lining in the periodontal pockets. This helps the gum tissues to heal).
- ☑ **Desensitizing of sensitive teeth** (applying a special seal to the tooth to prevent sensitivity).
- ☑ **Scaling** (removes the calculus deposits from your teeth).

☑ **Sub-gingival irrigation** (flushing below the gum margins with anti-microbial solution)

☑ Laser and Ozone desensitization and destruction of infective organisms

☑ Mouth-guards

☑ Orthodontics (teeth straightening) – using braces or retainers and positioners

☑ Pit and fissure sealants (mostly done for children; note that many sealants release BPA*s)

☑ Retainer & space maintainer

☑ Snoring and obstructive sleep apnea appliances

*Bisphenol A (BPA) is an industrial chemical used to make polycarbonate plastic resins, epoxy resins, and other products. It is used to make a variety of common consumer goods (such as baby and water bottles, sports equipment, CDs, and DVDs) and for industrial purposes, like lining water pipes. Epoxy resins containing BPA are used as coatings on the inside of many food and beverage cans. BPA exhibits hormone-like properties at high dosage levels that raise concern about its suitability in consumer products and food containers where exposure is orders of magnitude lower. The European Union and Canada have banned BPA use in baby bottles.

Part C: Symptoms of Mercury Toxicity

7. If you have any mercury fillings, commonly known as silver fillings, you need to assess their possible toxicity. This questionnaire* will assess how much damage has been done by the leaked mercury in your body.

The following questions will serve as a warning or to alert you. Please also refer to Chapter 4 to understand mercury fillings and some suggestions to detoxify their impact.

☒ Are you extremely fatigued much of the time and never seem to have enough energy?

☒ Are you on antidepressants now or have you been in the past?

☒ Do you crave alcohol or drugs?

☒ Do you have a lot of bad breath (halitosis) or a white coated tongue (thrush)?

☒ Do you have 'brown spots' or 'age spots' or dark circles under your eyes?

☒ Do you have heart irregularities or a rapid pulse (tachycardia)?

☒ Do you have irritability or dramatic changes in behaviour?

☒ Do you have numbness or burning sensations in your mouth or gums?

☒ Do you have numbness or unexplained tingling in your arms or legs?

☒ Do you have problems with constipation?

☒ Do you have ten or more mercury fillings?

☒ Do you have unexplained arthritis in various joints?

☒ Do you have unidentified chest pains even when ECG, x-ray and heart studies are normal?

☒ Do you often have a 'metallic' taste in your mouth?

☒ Has ringing in the ears (tinnitus) been present?

☒ Has severe depression been a frequent problem?

☒ Have TMJ (temporomandibular joint) problems been a concern?

☒ Have you been to many doctors, and they have usually said there is nothing wrong?

☒ Have you developed difficulty in walking (ataxia) over the years?

☒ Have you ever had Candida or yeast infections (vagina, mouth, or GI tract)?

☒ Have you ever worked as a painter or in factories (e.g. pulp/paper mills) that used mercury?

☒ Have you frequently had low basal body temperature, below 97.4 degrees F/ 36.5 degrees C?

☒ Have you had food allergies or intolerances?

☒ Have you had frequent kidney infections or do you have significant kidney problems?

☒ Have you had mental symptoms such as confusion, forgetfulness?

☒ Have you had sore gums (gingivitis) often over the years?

☒ Have you had unusual shakiness (tremors) of your hands or arms or twitching of muscles?

☒ Have you tended to have more colds, flu and other infectious diseases than 'normal'?

☒ Have you worked as a dentist or dental assistant?

☒ Is it common for you to have a lot of mucus in your stools?

☒ Is your sleep poor or do you have frequent insomnia?

*This questionnaire is part of a US FDA approved study called an Institutional Review Board.

> "Such questionnaires lead to a valid questioning of the toxic potential of mercury in your mouth, but NOT to the diagnosis of it. While some patients do seem to tolerate mercury in their mouth, others do not. A valid default position is a precautionary one - if it is in your mouth, consider removing it. If it is NOT in your mouth, don't put it there."
>
> - Dr. Brian McLean, DDS

You may also use the above questionnaires to assess general indication of your general health.

Details of a Survey of 1320 patients with mercury fillings are at

7stepsdentalhealth.com/?page_id=408

Details of a study of patients replacing the mercury fillings and their results are at 7stepsdentalhealth.com/?page_id=390

Part D: Your Routines and Lifestyle Issues

The following habits when done routinely will maintain ideal dental health. Yes to each of the questions indicates positive health.

8.   Educational Sessions

How many educational sessions or seminars have you attended and acted upon. These are preventive 'positive' steps to quality health.

- ☑ **Dietary nutritional supplement** recommendations for your teeth and body.
- ☑ Non-toxic oral hygiene product recommendations (as given in this book).
- ☑ Oral hygiene instruction (as given in this book).
- ☑ Reading dental books (such as this book).
- ☑ List any other educational sessions by dental health practitioners.

9.   Brushing

- ☑ Do you change your toothbrush at least, every three months?
- ☑ Do you brush your teeth after every meal or at least twice a day?
- ☑ Do you use a soft brush?
- ☑ Do you use an electric brush?
- ☑ You do not have any problem while brushing such as bleeding, sensitive teeth, irritation of the gums.
- ☑ Do you sanitize/sterilize your toothbrushes and tongue cleaners every week?

10. Flossing

- ☑ Do you floss your teeth (or practice Interdental cleaning) every night?
- ☑ You do not have any problem while flossing, such as bleeding, stuck floss between the teeth, sensitive teeth, irritation, etc.

11. Use of Dental Hygiene Products

   ☑ Do you rinse your teeth with a non-toxic mouthwash at least once a day?

   ☑ Do you have any problems (such as sensitive teeth, irritation of the gums) while using a mouthwash or toothpaste?

   ☑ Your toothpaste or mouthwash does not contain fluoride, SLS or other questionable ingredients as discussed in Chapter 3.

12. Food Habits

   ☑ Most of the time you eat healthy food (refer to Chapter 11 for Principles of Nutrition).

   ☑ You do not drink sodas/pop or sweet drinks.

   ☑ You do not eat snacks containing sugar.

   ☑ You drink enough water, filtered from chlorine and fluoride (six glasses are average for some, depending on your weight).

   ☑ You do not chew ice, candies or toffees.

   ☑ You do not smoke or chew tobacco.

   ☑ You do not consume alcohol.

   ☑ You do not suck on lemon or orange wedges.

Part E: Self- Examination Procedures for Oral Cancer

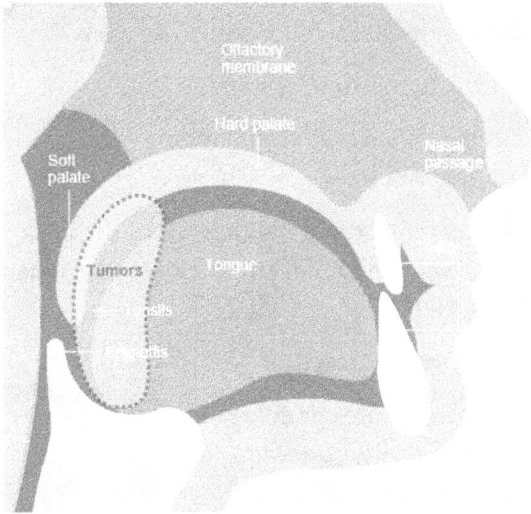

Cancer is defined as the uncontrollable growth of cells that invade and cause damage to surrounding tissue. Oral cancer is a group of cancers of the lips, tongue, cheeks, floor of the mouth, hard and soft palate, sinuses and pharynx (throat).

Oral cancer is the sixth most common cancer in the USA and affects twice as many men as women. Some of the risk factors of the oral cancer are tobacco products, alcohol, sunlight, lip biting, cheek biting, ill-fitting dentures, sharp or rough dental restorations and toxic chemicals, such as SLS.

Using a bright light and a mirror, perform the oral cancer self-examination; just follow these seven easy steps. Yes to each of the following assessments indicates poor health.

13.   Head and Neck - look at your face and neck in a mirror

   ☒   Normally, the left and right sides of the face have the same shape. Are yours symmetrical?

   ☒   Look for any lumps, bumps or swellings that are only on one side of your face.

14.   Face - examine the skin on your face

☒ Do you notice any colour or size changes in moles? Are they sore?

15.   Neck - press along the sides and front of the neck

☒ Do you feel any tenderness or lumps?

☒ Feel for lumps or enlarged lymph nodes on both sides of your neck and under your lower jaw.

☒ Do you feel any tightness along the side of the neck, which may be due to a slowdown of circulation and stagnation of the lymphatic glands?

16.   Lips - pull your lower lip down

☒ Look inside for any sores or colour changes. Use your thumb and forefinger to gently squeeze and roll the lip. Feel for lumps, bumps or changes in texture.

☒ Repeat this on your upper lip.

17.   Cheeks - use your fingers to pull out one cheek at a time, so you can see inside.

☒ Look for red, white, or dark patches or lines. Put your index finger on the inside of your cheek and your thumb on the outside. Gently squeeze and roll your cheek between your fingers to check for any lumps or areas of tenderness.

☒ Repeat this on the other cheek.

18.   Roof of the Mouth - tilt your head back and open your mouth wide to see it.

☒ Are there are any lumps or areas where the colour is different than usual.

☒ Run your finger on the roof to feel for lumps.

19.   Floor of the Mouth and Tongue

☒ Stick out your tongue and look at the top surface for colour and texture.

☒ Gently pull your tongue forward to look at one side first and then the other. Look for any swellings or colour changes.

☒ Examine the underside of your tongue by placing the tip of the tongue on the roof of your mouth. Can you see two strong purple lines or is one darker colour than the other line?

☒ Look at the floor of your mouth and the underside of your tongue for colour changes that are decidedly different from what is normal.

☒ Gently press your finger along the underside of your tongue to feel for any lumps or swellings.

If you find anything out of the ordinary and that does not heal or go away in two weeks, or that has recently changed, discuss it with your dental health professional or a physician.

To see photos of oral cancer symptoms visit the WebMD website at

www.webmd.com/oral-health/ss/slideshow-mouth-problems

Warning: Presence of any symptom or your assessment of any condition is subjective and not professional. The aim of self-assessment is to make you aware of the factors involved, but not to alarm you. You are strongly advised to take your assessment and any concerns to your dental and healthcare professionals.

CHAPTER 10

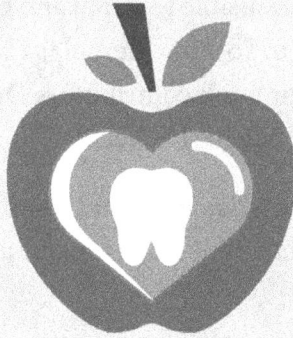

Dentistry in the Future

"The doctor of the future will give no medication, but will interest his patients in the care of the human frame, diet and in the cause and prevention of disease."

~ Thomas A. Edison

This chapter is based on available research and opinions of many health practitioners, such as Dr. Joseph Mercola, Carol Vander Stoep, Dr. Tim Rainey and from our book contributors Dr. Dana Colson, Dr. Iris Kivity-Chandler and Dr. Michael Schecter.

Please note that equipment, technologies and trends mentioned in this section are not endorsed by the authors and contributors and some of them may be controversial.

This Chapter has three Sections:

1. Future Trends in Dentistry
2. Advancements in Diagnostics and Restorations
3. My Wish List for Dental Practice

Section1:
Future Trends in Dentistry

Here are some innovative procedures, trends, and technology, which I believe will be common place soon. They are given below in alphabetical order:

Air Abrasion

During *air abrasion*, a fine stream of particles is aimed at the stained or decayed portion of the tooth. These particles are made of silica, aluminium oxide, or a baking soda mixture and are propelled toward the tooth surface by compressed *air* or a gas that runs through the *dental* hand piece.

Biomimetic Dentistry (BD)

Tooth preservation and dental conservation lie at the heart of biomimetic dentistry. Biomimetic dentistry, a type of "tooth conserving dentistry", treats weak, fractured, and decayed teeth in a way that keeps them strong and seals them from bacterial invasion. In dental practices around the world, Biomimetic Dentistry has practically eliminated the practice of cutting teeth down for crowns and destructive root canal treatment. Patients are happier and often spend less money compared to conventional treatment.

Biomimetic dentistry offers excellent alternatives to large fillings and crowns, such as inlays, onlays and crowns. These are permanent restorations that do not need to be replaced with restorations like regular resin fillings and metal or porcelain crowns. BD means 'mimicking nature', and involves using tooth restorations and techniques *that imitate natural teeth, both in appearance and function.*

Dental Revision

Dental revision involves removing toxic stressors of oral origin, such as dead teeth, dead jawbone, metal teeth restorations, and meridian-blocking implants.

Advancements in Diagnostics (detailed in the next section)

There are some areas where advanced diagnostics can help in preserving tooth, such as:

- Diagnosing vitality in the teeth if a tooth requires a root canal.
- Diagnosing necrotic bone in an extraction site or around a previous root canal treated tooth.

- Non-Invasive Diagnostics: We will see rapid improvements in diagnostics tools, some integrated with existing digital radiography and intraoral cameras. Some specific equipment are outlined in the next section

Eliminating Sedation

A number of techniques will be explored such, such as:

- Use of laser without the need for local anaesthesia

- Hypnosis

- Meditation

- Reiki

Making Crowns (detailed in the next section)

A dentist will be able to make crowns, denture or bridges in the clinic by using scanners and digital modelling (like 3-D printers).

Minimally Invasive Dentistry (MID)

The act of drilling into a tooth is destructive to the tooth, especially when using a high speed drill. It can create tiny little cracks that lead to further deterioration of the tooth over time. Low-speed drilling is not as destructive to the tooth but is still far from optimal. The conventional strategy to "drill and fill," regardless of the restorative material used, is not a permanent solution. An estimated 70-80 percent of the work done by dentists involves re-repairing previous dental work. MID offers dramatically safer and more effective solutions.

The concept of minimally invasive dentistry is still in its infancy, although Dr. Tim Rainey, adjunct associate professor at the University of Texas Health Science Center School of Dentistry, has been tirelessly lecturing on the subject, all over the world, for the last twenty-five years.

Lasers (detailed in the next section)

Lasers have been used in dentistry for more than twenty-years. We have gone from treating only soft tissue to treating hard tissues such as teeth and bone. The cost of soft-tissue lasers has decreased along with their size. General dentists can now easily integrate lasers into their practices.

Some specific dental lasers, such as the diode laser and Nd:YAG are being used in North America. These lasers are being used in non-surgical periodontal treatment regimens by removing the diseased epithelial lining of the periodontal pocket and reducing the intrasulcular bacterial population.

The Canadian Academy of Periodontology (CAP) and the American Academy of Periodontology (AAP) do not support the use of lasers in the treatment of periodontal disease due to the lack of long-term comparative studies.

Nanodentistry/ Nanorobotics in Dentistry

Nanotechnology is based on the concept of creating functional structures by controlling atoms and molecules on a one-by-one basis. The use of this technology will allow many developments in the health sciences. Nanotechnology can be used for various procedures, such as:

- Local anaesthesia
- Dentition renaturalization
- Cure for hypersensitivity
- Complete orthodontic realignment in a single visit
- Covalently bonded diamondized enamel
- Continuous oral health maintenance
- Dental Nano robots could be constructed to destroy caries-causing bacteria
- Repair tooth blemishes where decay has set in

Orthodontics

Advances in technology have produced bracket and wire systems such as Damon by Ormco, which make the treatment more comfortable, more aesthetically pleasing and take less time consuming.

Clear aligners, are orthodontic devices that use incremental transparent aligners to adjust teeth as an alternative to dental braces. In particular they are indicated for moderate crowding. These slowly move the teeth into the position agreed between the dentist and the patient. Clear aligners can replace Damon brackets.

TADs, (Temporary Anchorage Devices). Orthodontists are accustomed to using teeth and auxiliary appliances, both intraoral and extra oral, to control anchorage. These methods are limited in that it is often difficult to achieve desired results. Recently, a number of case reports have appeared in the orthodontic literature documenting the possibility of overcoming anchorage limitations via the use of temporary anchorage devices—biocompatible devices fixed to bone for the purpose of moving teeth, with the devices being subsequently removed after treatment.

Jaw joints, airways, posture, the quality of sleep are evaluated to understand causes of malocclusion (imperfect positioning of the teeth when the jaws are closed).

Ozone (O$_3$)

Ozone, an energized form of oxygen, is a proven potent anti-microbial and anti-inflammatory agent. As a gas, it can penetrate easily and with a strong negative charge, ozone gets pulled like a magnet towards the infection. Ozone is 5000 times more effective than chlorine. Ozone can be viewed as an amplification of our own natural defence. White blood cells produce ozone to combat disease.

Ozone is very effective in dentistry. Ozone can disinfect root canals and fillings. It can be used to prevent and treat infections that may occur after surgery. The highly unstable ozone molecule (O3) wants desperately to kick off one oxygen, so it can return to the more stable O2 molecule. According to book, *Ozone, the Dental Revolution* by Dr. Ed Lynch and Dr. Julian Holmes:

"Powerful reaction drives oxygen beneath the surface of a tooth through the tubules and kill bacteria in early decay and it essentially start a process that removes bacterial waste products, halts dental cavities, and begins a process of repair via accelerated remineralization."

Prevention of Disease

Dentist approach will be education and prevention followed by restoration and treatment. Technology will make the education accessible and available before and after the dental office visits.

Regenerative Procedures

Procedures that regenerate lost bone and tissue supporting your teeth can reverse some of the damage caused by periodontal disease. A number of techniques are used to achieve that, such as:

- Removing the disease-causing bacteria by folding back the gum tissue.
- Encouraging body's natural ability to regenerate bone and tissue by procedures like Membranes (filters), bone grafts or tissue-stimulating proteins.
- Nd:Yag or CO2 lasers can also help regeneration case specific.

Robotics in Dentistry

A dental robot was created to perform dental procedures at the 79th General Session of the International Association for Dental Research in 2001. The field has advanced and one day we will see robots doing routine dentistry tasks. Robotics will also allow dentists to operate from a distance at a remote location.

Salivary Diagnostics for General Conditions

Saliva is a clear, slightly acidic (pH = 6.0-7.0) watery fluid which is secreted from the major salivary glands, including the parotid, submandibular, and sublingual glands in addition to other minor glands. It contains a variety of enzymes, hormones, antibodies, antimicrobial constituents, and cytokines.

Saliva has been progressively studied as a non-invasive and relatively stress-free diagnostic alternative to blood. Saliva is now being used to detect a growing number of oral diseases:

- Caries
- Periodontal disease
- Oral cancer
- Systemic disorders

Short Time-frame to Implement Research

Medicine and Dental practice lag behind in catching up with advances and research. Some of the current practices have taken as much as two decades to be implemented. Due to advances in the communication we have today the gap will become shorter.

Stem cells Applicability in Dentistry

Stem cells have the potential to repair and regenerate teeth and periodontal structures. These stem cells can be harvested from dental pulp, periodontal ligament, and/or alveolar bone marrow. These stem cells can be embedded in an appropriate scaffold and transplanted back into a defect to regenerate bone and tooth structures.

Workflow in Dentistry

Over the next few years digital dentistry will profoundly change the way dentists will treat patients, work with the laboratory, and store the patient's intra oral records. Digital dental technology is an integration of many technologies and advancements in dentistry in general and implant in particular, such as:

- Digital data acquisition
- Comprehensive virtual implant treatment planning
- Digital designing of surgical guides
- CAD/CAM guided surgery
- Digital restorative approaches
- CAD/CAM restoration manufacturing
- 3-D radiographic/photographic imaging
- Guided surgery
- Intra-oral digital impressions
- Chair side milling of provisional restorations
- Construction of a surgical guide for guided surgery
- Digital design and fabrication of implant borne restorations

Some of them are highlighted in this section while others appear in the next section. Hopefully dentists will explore and implement new ideas and technologies.

Section 2:
Advancements in Diagnostics and Treatment

Technology is advancing at a rapid pace, and dental professionals are now able to serve patients in ways that could not have been imagined just a few years ago. Dental technology today is truly astounding.

We will also explore some innovative technologies, which are not new but are not prevalent in use. This happens in medicine and dentistry for a number of reasons, such as controversy, the need to achieve a different chairside outcome or expense. An example of such technology is T-Scan (see below) which was invented in 1987 but not widely used. There are several other such technologies appearing in the market that improves the ability to detect biofilm, inflammation, and dental caries, such as SoproCARE. Unfortunately, dentists, like other professionals, take a long time to implement new and innovative technologies.

3D Printing Makes the Digital Physical

Instead of the dentist receiving the same green stone model for over thirty years, what if a lifelike full colour model showed the difference in the teeth and gum tissue? Or a model that allowed you to see complete tooth and nerve anatomy? Better than any digital Photoshop-like simulation allows one to hold a full colour replica of their teeth with a 3D printed version.

AlfaSight 9000.

AlfaSight 9000 is a tool to detect infections from root canal and caviatation. The **AlfaSight 9000** is a non-invasive patient assessment tool that identifies a wide range of physiological dysfunction by analysing skin temperature fluctuations over time. As an adjunct technology to mammography and other anatomical imaging devices, it can dramatically improve the accuracy of routine testing for a wide range of impaired health conditions.

Alternative Treatment Modalities

There has been explosion of various testing and diagnostics tools in alternative medicine, such as *iridology, bio-impedance testing, hair analysis, applied kinesiology, meridian analysis, oxidative stress measurement and as well as a broader movement toward patient self-empowerment, self-care and personal responsibility.*

Anaesthetic Buffering 2.0

A common buffering agent used for anaesthetic is sodium bicarbonate, a chemical that is difficult to keep stable, for the entire duration of the operation / procedure. The idea has now been refined with Anutra local anaesthetic delivery system.

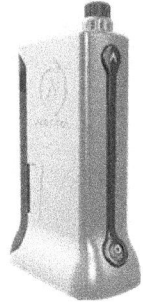

Cavitat

A cavitation is a hole in the bone, often where a tooth has been removed and the bone has not filled in properly. In the last several years, the term cavitation has been used to describe various bone lesions which appear both as empty holes in the jawbones and holes filled with dead bone and bone marrow.

There is a technology that has been developed that can image the jaw bone using unfocused ultrasound. It provides a colour-coded three dimensional representation of the density of the bone and shows loss of bone or ischemic dying bone tissue that is usually not seen on x-ray imaging. This technology, called a Cavitat, has been approved by the FDA and is now available. It has an incredibly high accuracy record in the findings of a correctly performed scan.

CEREC (CEramic REConstruction)

The CEREC system lets your dentist provide a ceramic crown or veneer in only one visit. CEREC means fewer injections, less drilling and no annoying temporaries. CEREC is like a use of robotics in dentistry. It is a combination of machines (scanning/camera unit – milling unit) allowing the dentist to produce an immediate restoration in a single visit.

Dental cone beam computed tomography (CT)

It is a special type of x-ray equipment *used* when regular *dental* or facial x-rays are not sufficient. Your doctor may *use* this technology to produce three dimensional (3-D) images of your teeth, soft tissues, nerve pathways and bone in a single scan. The technology has been available and will become more prevalent.

Dental digital impression systems

These high tech systems simplify the impression process, increase accuracy, decrease procedure time and enable digital integration with dental laboratories. Digital impressions eliminate the technique sensitivity and patient discomfort of using impression materials, and the 3D digital models they create are highly accurate and detailed. Captured using safe, non-invasive imaging technologies, digital impressions are available for a range of restorative and orthodontic dental situations. The scans are ready almost instantly and can be sent directly to a dental lab or to a chairside CAD/CAM system without the need to pour a model.

Dental Intraoral X-ray Sensors

These have been shown to be every bit as diagnostic as film radiographs, while offering clinicians a lot more when it comes to diagnostics and ways the images can be used. With better resolution, dramatically reduced radiation to the patient, and the ability to zoom into parts of the image as well as used filters for enhanced diagnostics, digital dental X-ray systems are friendlier to the patient, and to the doctor. Add to that the ability to archive radiographs with no loss of image quality, as well as the ability to send a perfect digital copy to insurance companies or referral partners.

Dental Practice Management Software

Dental Practice Management Software serves as the hub of the modern dental practice, such as a Toronto software, Velo Mobile Health, even facilitates sending reminders (email, text, etc.) to patient's smart phones and their response automatically, saving valuable staff time and ensuring patient communication.

Diagnodent

Diagnodent is a laser that the dentist shines on the tooth and it tells whether there is a cavity and how deep it is. With the use of this technology, the dentist can detect some cavities, and find them at an earlier stage, rather than using the traditional method of examining the tooth.

EAV (Electro Acupuncture according to Voll)/ Electrodermal Screening (EDS)

An EKG measures the electrical flow through your heart. Expressed as a graph, it pinpoints heart damage, since current does not flow through dead tissues. EAV works the same way. The EAV test uses an ohmmeter to measure the energy flow along meridians at acupuncture points. If you understand meridians and you've signed on to "Healing is Voltage," "The Body Electric" and understand the science behind "Earthing", you know low-functioning organs are low in negative ions.

This state hinders electron flow along your body's energy meridians. Dr. WA Tiller, Professor Emeritus of Materials Science at Stanford University, set out to discredit the EAV, but became an advocate as his research verified organ degeneration correlated with low conductance. In fact, it was Dr. Tiller, who mapped the Meridian Tooth Chart, which correlates each tooth with its associated organs, glands, and anatomical structures on the same meridian. Infected or diseased teeth, as well as dental implants, block the electrical conductivity on meridians and so can alter the health of other organs located on the same meridian and vice versa.

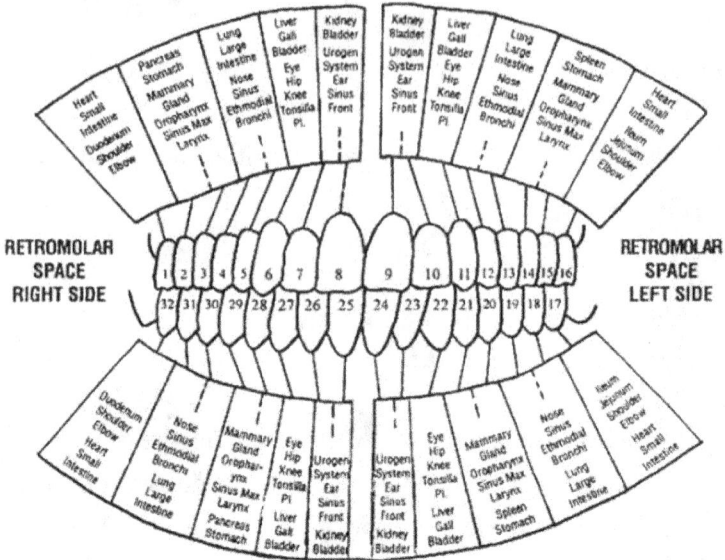

Details http://toothbody.com/learning-center/meridian-tooth-chart/

Galileos 3-D Scanner

This scanner generates a 3D image after only fourteen seconds, providing an exceptionally high image resolution in a short period of time. This means less waiting time for a diagnosis and treatment plans.

Implants Keep Improving

Dental implants have been around for decades, but we continue to see tweaks to systems on the surgical side, as well as restorative connections. Many companies have advanced various connectors to follow the internal conical connection that has shown success, and has introduced straight, non-tapered implants with that connection. These implants also have ability to place the access hole at an angle.

Lasers: The Technology that Continually Redefines Itself

Lasers have emerged with an ever expanded list of procedures using a dental laser, especially in periodontics.

Below are a few laser devices:

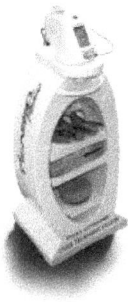

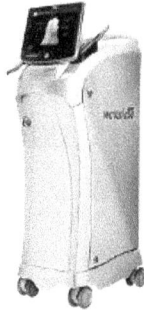

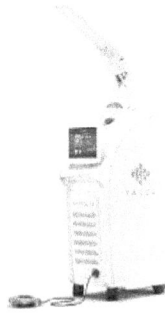

AMD Lasers brought their diode laser into the perio space with the new Picasso Perio Dental laser. The tiny laser sits on top of a cart designed to be an all-in-one station for perio treatment.

WaterLase iPlus 2.0 by BIOLASE. Designed for cutting hard and soft tissue, this erbium laser also comes with on-board settings for various perio indications which can help guide a clinician through the laser perio treatments.

CO2 laser, Solea by Convergent Dental also for hard and soft tissue. The Ultraguide hand piece and 15/400 Hollow Waveguide are designed to deliver the 0.25 mm beam into the pocket for treatment of Perio disease and periimplantitis.

The Canary System is a precise, low-powered, laser-based instrument with an integrated intraoral camera that detects the presence of cracks and caries (tooth decay) before they are large enough to appear on dental X-rays. Intraoral camera images can be displayed for immediate chair side review with the patient. A patient report is generated containing an odontogram with Canary Numbers, which are colour-coded for the examined teeth, along with the dentist's treatment recommendation. This report can also be examined by the patient on The Canary Cloud

SoproCARE: intraoral camera

ACTEON North America has developed a high-performance intraoral camera that can highlight dental plaque, gingival inflammation, and effectively assists in enamo-dentinal caries detection. The camera utilizes unique fluorescence technology (SOPRO patent* – 2003) to illuminate dental tissue to reveal caries in CARIO mode, as well as new and old dental plaque in PERIO mode.

The camera is unique in that it has 3 modes.

1. It has a Daylight mode for natural high quality image of the tissues.

2. CARIO mode that uses the blue light to amplify the fluorescent chroma for visual detection of dental caries.

3. PERIO mode that combines the blue and white lights to highlight any biofilm and inflammation that may be present (Figures 3 and 4).

T-Scan to improve Dental Occlusion

Dental occlusion refers to the way your teeth meet when you bite together. Your teeth should come in contact with one another at the same time and with equal force. When this doesn't occur your occlusion is unbalanced which may cause many problems. It is a diagnostic device that measures relative biting forces, including occlusal force, timing and location, and it is an ideal complement to articulating paper. The technology was invented by Dr. William Maness in 1987 at Tufts University and M.I.T.

Thermographics

Some tools are available, but they are not integrated in the dental practice, such as a traditional camera-imaged thermogram (used for detecting early stage breast cancer). Thermographic images display infrared heat emissions, with each colour gradation indicating different heat emissions. High-heat emissions are suggestive of inflammation, which may indicate root canal toxicity or a cavitation—even if you're without any symptoms.

Section 3:
Max Haroon's Wish List for Dental Practice

Technology is evolving at an exponential rate. The advent of technology will bring efficiency to the dental practice and it should bring the dental treatment cost down. Below is the Author's wishful thinking:

1.   **Start with Dental Exam & Remove Toxicity:** No matter what health condition you may have, get your oral assessment and remove any dental infection and toxicity. When you are not healthy not only it will be reflected in your mouth, but it could be the cause of it. My hope is that hospitals and other treatment centres to adopt this protocol, which is currently practiced by Hippocrates Institute, where the patient goes through a thorough oral exam and dental detox before commencing any treatment.

2.   **Patient-centric:** My hope is that medicine and dentistry will be patient centric. The patient should be able to participate fully in the process of diagnostics and treatment. This is only possible if the dentist becomes a partner in the process and provides education when required.

3.   **Detox and Nutrition:** Dentist will have enough knowledge about nutrition and detoxification to advise patients to detoxify from heavy metals (mercury, lead, etc.). Research has indicated that removal of these toxins is imperative for treatment.

4.   **Mercury-free dentistry:** Dentists will stop using mercury and overall dentistry will become mercury-free. Although many countries have banned mercury filling, North America's dental

associations plus health agencies (such as FDA, Health Canada) are secretive about the use of mercury in dental practice (I am wondering who is stopping these organizations from banning mercury!) I would like to see a complete ban on mercury use, or any metal use, for restoration work.

5. **Affordability:** Dentists will provide dental care to those who cannot afford it. As shown in the stats only 40% of the population receives dental care, and 98% need it. Unfortunately, 60% do not have the money or desire to see a dentist. My hope for the future is that dentists will not gouge the patients for exorbitant and sometime unnecessary/unwarranted treatments.

6. **Holistic approach:** In the future, I would like to see dentists and hygienists employ a holistic approach to therapies and treatment. Biological dentistry views your teeth and gums as an integrated part of your entire body as such for any treatment, he /she should consider its impact on the whole body. He or she should be concerned about sleep apnea, jaw-related pain known as TMJ (temporomandibular joint) disorder, periodontal disease, oral cancer, diabetes and hypertension.

7. **Education and Prevention:** My wish for the future is that dental offices become a hub of patient education. All health practitioners claim that believe in the prevention of disease, however their practice is traditional. I would like all practitioners to believe in it and practice prevention by allocating some resources to it.

8. **Biocompatible materials:** Dentists use biocompatible materials that will not adversely impact your immune system.

9. **Anaesthetic injections:** It is my wish that dentists will introduce protocols that would reduce discomfort. Or if available, protocol to reduce injections altogether. Many such methods are available for example: hypnosis, Reiki and other anti-anxiety protocols.

10. **Dental & Other Specialists:** It will be synergistic to have specialists such as osteopaths, nutritionist, naturopaths, Homeopaths and Reiki Masters under one roof. There are some dental clinics where you will see a blend of such practices, such as Schecter Dental and Dana Colson & Associates, but they are few and far between. The dentist should call upon other specialist as

part of his service rather than patients having to see and pay for them separately.

11. **Alternatives to Root Canal Procedure:** A root canal is an embalming procedure dentists perform on a tooth. Root canals are designed to keep a dead tooth mechanically functioning in a live body. Dentists will focus in maintaining the vitality in teeth, so that root canal procedures are minimised.

12. **All dentists to follow the six principles of classical medicine:**

The underpinnings of Naturopathic medical practice are in six principles:

- *primum non nocere* - First, Do No Harm

- *vis medicatrix naturae* – The Healing Power of Nature

- *tolle causam* - Discover and Treat the Cause, Not Just the effect

- *tolle totum* - Treat the Whole Person

- *docere* - The Physician is a Teacher

- *praevenire* - Prevention is the best "cure"

CHAPTER 11

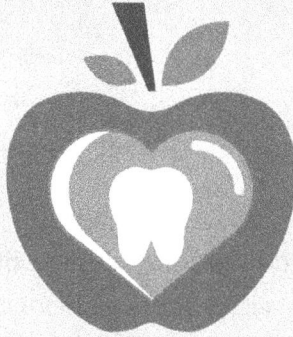

Food and Nutrition
for Dental Health

"Let food be thy medicine and medicine be thy food"
~ Hippocrates 460 - 359 BC

Teeth are just one part of the human body. Any imbalance and stress, in any part of the body, including the teeth, disturb the overall health of the body.

In order to provide strength and nourishment to the teeth, the body needs to be nourished.

In this chapter, we will focus on essential nourishment and nutrition - food, vitamins, minerals and nutritional supplements.

By not paying attention to what we eat, how we eat, and our lifestyle, we have developed chronic diseases such as gum disorders, cardiovascular disease, blood pressure imbalance, diabetes, obesity and thyroid imbalance.

Why do we need food?

- The simple answer is we eat because we are hungry; we are hungry because we need energy and food is the main source of energy.
- Food rebuilds tissues in our body. About 98% of the body is completely remade this way in a year. You are what you eat, so if you want a healthier you then you should eat healthy food.
- Food fights inflammation and build immunity, so we need food to heal.

Some of the food characteristics and categories you should pay attention in order to understand the science behind food.

Next time when you look at food, consider many of its characteristics:
- Alkalinity and Acidity
- Glycemic Index/Glycemic Load
- Organic* (see below)
- Sugar Content
- Fibre Content
- Compatibility with your gut/allergy/intolerance

Section 1:
Glycemic Index (GI) & Fibre

Glycemic Index (GI)

A newer Index called Glycemic Load (GL) measures the amount of carbohydrate in each serving (portion size) of food. The GL provides a reliable tool for the management of diabetes and obesity.

The Glycemic Index (GI) is a measure of how quickly foods raise blood glucose (on a scale from 0 to 100). High GI foods turn into glucose very quickly (which is not suitable for you), while Low GI foods turn into glucose slowly.

- High GI Foods (GI 70 or more) e.g., potatoes, ice cream, white flour
- Intermediate GI Foods (GI 55-69) e.g., oatmeal cookie, orange juice, white rice
- Low GI Foods (GI 54 or less) e.g., rice bran, oat bran, apples, berries, most vegetables and nuts

Check out the GI Index of Various Foods www.trans4mind.com/nutrition/glycemic_index.html

Pioneering work by David Jenkins, a U of T Researcher was published in the book, "*The G.I. Factor*". Published later as "The *New Glucose Revolution*", 2003. www.mendosa.com/gifactor.htm

GL Index of Some Foods

A newer Index called Glycemic Load (GL) measures the amount of carbohydrate in each serving (portion size) of food. The GL provides a reliable tool for the management of diabetes and obesity.

Notice, for each food in the example below, a serving size is given in parentheses. GL Index of 19 or below is considered good for you.

- Low GL (10 or under) is best, such as:

Fish (150 gm) is 0, chickpeas (80 gm) are 4, and berries (120 gm) are 0.

- Medium GL (11-19) is good, such as:

  Spaghetti (180 gm) is 17; honey (25 gm) is 10.

- High GL (20 plus) is bad, such as:

  Corn flakes, white rice, dates, raisins, condensed milk, pearl barley, pop tarts, bran muffins, canned pea soup, gluten-free corn pasta.

Check out the GI and GL of Various Foods at Glycemic Index (GI) and Glycemic Load (GL) Values. www.mendosa.com/gilists.htm

An excellent source of the Glycemic Index and Glycemic Load for 100+ foods is available at Harvard Health Publications www.health.harvard.edu/newsweek/Glycemic_index_and_glycemic_load_for_100_foods.htm

Fibre

Low GL foods are also high in fibre, so select foods that fall between 10 and 20 on the Glycemic Load. If you do eat foods with a Glycemic Load above 20 then compensate its glucose load by supplementing with soluble fibre.

If you think you have an overdose of sugar and other toxic load, then consider cleansing the body by detoxification. Start by taking lots of fibre.

Metabolic conditions like obesity, diabetes, pre-diabetes and other chronic diseases relate to the body's ability to handle glucose and its storage.

Soluble fibre in the foods binds cholesterol in the digestive system, so the cholesterol is unable to get into the blood circulation. Therefore, by increasing the fibre you are detoxifying and lowering the bad cholesterol.

Americans eat 5 to 20 gm of fibre a day. Dieticians recommend 25 – 30 gm of fibre per day, or six to ten gm per meal. Each of the following foods provides approximately 10 gm of mixed fibre (soluble and insoluble):

- ½ cup lentils or split peas
- 1 cup elderberries or blackberries
- 1 tsp xanthan gum

- 1 cup flax seed
- 3 Tbsp psyllium seed
- *1 ounce oat or wheat bran*

Section 2:
Alkaline and Acidic Foods

Food is classified as alkaline, acid or neutral according to its residue when burned into fuel after its consumption and absorption into the blood.

If the residue is alkaline-ash, mostly consisting of calcium, potassium, sodium, magnesium, zinc, it is classified as alkaline.

If the residue is acidic-ash, such as phosphorus then the food is classified as acidic. All foods and drinks leave either an alkaline-ash or acid-ash in the blood.

Acidic Foods

- Sugar
- Proteins, cereals, grains, beans and dairy
- Stimulants like tobacco, coffee, black & green tea, and alcohol
- Most manufactured processed foods
- Some fruit like cranberries

Stress, fear and worry also cause acidification. Stress plays a major part in weakening your immune system, thus making you susceptible to getting sick.

Alkaline Foods

- Water with a good salt - alkaline water
- Most fruit
- Most vegetables and vegetable soups

- Herbs, spices and herbal teas
- Water with lemon juice

It is necessary to consume at least 60% alkaline-producing foods in your diet in order to maintain health. We need to avoid processed, sugary or simple carbohydrate foods, not only because they are acid-producing but also because they raise blood sugar levels too quickly.

Acidosis will decrease the body's ability to absorb minerals and other nutrients, decrease the energy production in cells, decrease its ability to repair damaged cells, decrease its ability to detoxify heavy metals, make tumour cells thrive, and make you more susceptible to fatigue and illness. It also decreases the assimilation of vitamins, minerals and food supplements.

Say no to most of the acidic foods such as white sugar, white flour, and boxed cereals. According to some dietician milk is slightly acidic while goat's milk is not.

pH Measurement

Alkalinity or acidity is measured on a pH scale 0 to 14. Less than seven is acidic, and more than seven is alkaline,

7 pH is neutral. Human blood pH should be slightly alkaline (7.35 - 7.45).

If blood pH moves below 6.8 or above 7.8, the cells stop functioning, and the body dies.

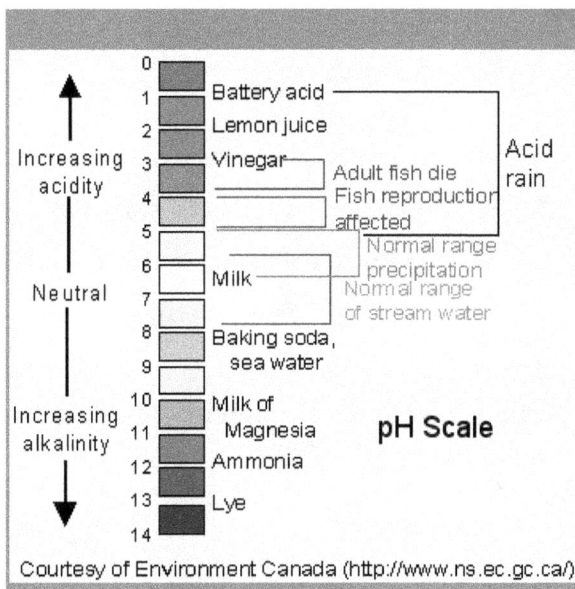

Increasing acidity

0
1 Battery acid
2 Lemon juice
3 Vinegar — Adult fish die   Acid rain
4   Fish reproduction affected
5
6 Milk   Normal range precipitation
Neutral 7   Normal range of stream water
8 Baking soda,
9   sea water
10 Milk of
Increasing alkalinity 11   Magnesia   **pH Scale**
12 Ammonia
13 Lye
14

Courtesy of Environment Canada (http://www.ns.ec.gc.ca/)

Alkaline and Acid forming food chart www.trans4mind.com/nutrition/pH.html

The body will titrate (to alter the pH to acceptable level) acidic substances before allowing them into blood plasma. If minerals not available from the GI tract, to alter pH level, it will take calcium from the bones to raise blood pH. If chronic condition (done in continuing basis) will lead to osteoporosis.

High GI foods are also acidic and damage the inside of the arteries (an inflammatory condition). When chronic, inflammatory proteins are produced by the immune system which will become systemic and can attack other areas of your body where you are vulnerable. A condition in the arteries called glycation can also occur which does damage by causing bleeding and creating clots.

Phil Feilds, Wellness Educator

Section 3:
Holistic Food

A dietary regimen based on the nourishing traditions involves eating whole grains and protein in balance with fats, seeds, herbs and spices. Weston A. Price found, in his travels in the 1930's, that tribes with perfectly white, straight teeth ate a diet of 20% protein, 40% fat, and 40% carbohydrates.

www.westonaprice.org/basics/dietary-guidelines

We can learn a lot from these principles as they are as historical as stated by Hippocrates, the father of Western Medicine. Hufeland, a German physician, in his book *Makrobiotik, The Art of Prolonging Life*, 1797, first used the word "macrobiotics" in the context of food and health.

Whole Food Principles

Whole food principles for both Macrobiotic and Holistic philosophies are remarkably similar. They are outlined below:

- Choosing food that is less processed.

- Becoming aware of the actual effects of foods on the body and well-being, rather than following dietary rules and regulations.

- Locally grown organic and seasonal food is preferred.

- Recommends against overeating.

- Food should be chewed thoroughly before swallowing.

- Periodic fasting is advisable.

Micronutrients Available in Holistic Food

Some foods contain the following micronutrients:

- Calcium & magnesium are available from hard leafy greens, nuts and seeds.

- Zinc is available from nuts and seeds.

- Fish provides vitamin B12 as bioavailable B12.

- Vitamin A, in the form of beta-carotene.

- Sources of Omega-3 fatty acids include soy products, walnuts, pumpkin seeds, flax seeds and fatty fish.

- Riboflavin, along with most other B vitamins, is abundant in whole grains.

- Iron in the form of non-heme iron is found in beans, sea vegetables and leafy greens.

"In addition to holistic food, we also need emotional, spiritual, relationship and environmental nourishment; in other words we need Holistic Nourishment for Holistic Well-being".

Max Haroon, Founder, Life Transformation Institute

Section 4:
Artificial Sweeteners
and Sugar Replacements

Artificial Sweeteners

Artificial chemical sweeteners like saccharin and aspartame are created in laboratories and have no business being in a human body. These super sweet crystals are synthetic chemicals with a sweet taste, but, in a few cases, they have been linked to a variety of serious, even life-threatening illnesses.

Examples of such products: Sweet' N Low, Equal, NutraSweet.

Try to avoid heavily processed foods with artificial colours, sweeteners and chemicals, such as:

- Aspartame (found in NutraSweet, Equal)
- Acesulfame potassium (found in Sunett, Sweet One)
- Neotame (used in commercial food products)
- Sodium saccharin/saccharin (found in Sweet' N Low, Sugar Twin)
- Sucralose (found in Splenda, Nevella)
- MSG (Mono Sodium Glutamate)

Research shows that MSG is a neurotoxin damaging to the nervous system or brain, linked to hormonal imbalances, weight gain, obesity and a variety of other health problems.

Eat more certified organic fruit and vegetables that are grown without herbicide, sprayed pesticide, radiation and chemical fertilizers.

Read the books:

"Hard to Swallow" and *"ASPARTAME (NutraSweet) Is it Safe?*

Books about Medical, Environmental & Pharmaceutical Systems

life-transformation-institute.org/resources/books/environment_
health_books.htm

Sugar Replacements

Many people these days live a healthier lifestyle. They reduce refined, deadly white table sugar and replace it with the following:

- Stevia
- Xylitol
- Unrefined Cane sugar (Sucanat)

Stevia (Rebaudiana)

There are nearly 300 species of the stevia family scattered over the region extending from the southwestern United States to northern Argentina. Stevia rebaudiana is a small shrub native to portions of Northeastern Paraguay and adjacent regions of Brazil. South American natural scientist Antonio Bertoni first "discovered" it in 1887, while native Indians from the Guarani Tribe have used it as a sweetener since pre-Columbian times.

The sweet secret of stevia lies in a complex molecule called stevioside, which is a glucoside, composed of glucose, sophorose and steviol. It is this complex molecule and a number of other related compounds that account for stevia rebaudiana's extraordinary sweetness. It is between 100 and 300 times sweeter than white table sugar.

Traditionally, it is being used as a sweetener, but is also used as medicine, in cosmetics, personal care ingredients and in toothpastes. Stevia has become a major export crop and is now cultivated in over a dozen industrialized countries. The largest user is Japan after they banned certain artificial sweeteners in the late sixties and it increased its usage due to the health concerns of Japanese consumers toward sucrose as it related to dental decay, obesity and diabetes. Stevioside has also been approved as a food additive in South Korea, China, Taiwan and Malaysia, Brazil and Paraguay.

Xylitol

Xylitol is another safe alternative to sugar; it is derived from certain fruits, vegetables, berries, nut shells, birch wood, corn residues, straw and seed hulls. It has no known propensity to cause decay. In fact, regular use of Xylitol-containing products, such as toothpaste, gums, candies, lozenges and others, can halt tooth decay in its tracks and may even promote the healing of cavities that are already underway. If young children are using products that include Xylitol, as long as they take care of their teeth, they may be protected against decay for the rest of their lives.

Xylitol interferes with the bacteria that cause tooth decay, halting their growth and preventing them from sticking to tooth surfaces. It is ideal for children, because Xylitol sweetened foods taste just as enjoyable as those sweetened with sucrose. Serious anti-decay research using Xylitol goes back more than 25 years. In a recent research, Dr. Catherine Hayes of the Harvard School of Dental Medicine concluded that the favourable evidence for Xylitol was so strong that it would be unethical to deprive people of its dental protective effects.

Xylitol is toxic to dogs, so be careful if you have a dog in the house, even chewing gum with Xylitol can be deadly for dogs.

Dental Benefits of Xylitol & Videos about Xylitol, www.xylitol.org/xylitol-videos

Cane Sugar

Cane sugar is extracted from the sugarcane, a tropical plant that produces naturally high concentrations of this sweet substance. Humans have been utilizing cane sugar in cooking for more than 150 years, and cane sugar was at one point and still today, a major element in global trade.

Today, most markets carry cane sugar in a variety of forms, from minimally processed, raw, dark brown sugar to white sugar cubes. Cane sugar typically tends to be a more expensive form of sucrose, but many people prefer it because they think it has a superior flavour.

As early as 3000 BCE, people in India were crushing the stalks to make juice and then evaporating the juice to create sugar crystals. Throughout Southeast Asia and the Middle East, cane sugar was used for centuries before it was introduced to Europe, where honey had been the only sweetener available. Shortly before 1000 BC, sugar cane was under cultivation in Spain, and the Spanish brought sugarcane with them to their Caribbean colonies, where it became a linchpin in the so-called "Triangular Trade" of slaves, sugar and rum.

Please remember - cane sugar is still a sugar.

Section 5:
Recommendations

In addition to various characteristics pay attention to the following factors:

- What to eat and what not to eat
- When to eat and when not to eat
- How to eat and how to avoid eating in certain situations
- How much and how little to eat
- What to eat with what and what to avoid eating certain foods with other foods
- Characteristics of food

It is not the intention of this book to be a nutrition manual, but rather to bring together new and old findings with my perspective on the subject of nutrition.

Food and nutrition alone will not give you total health. Lifestyle, environment and genetics also play a vital part.

Food is not only fuel for your body, but it provides essential nourishment and antioxidants (ingredients that fight free radicals in your body. Free radicals cause many illnesses).

*Organic food is grown without synthetic pesticides, insecticides, herbicides, fungicides, hormones, fertilizers or other synthetic or toxic substances. No artificial flavours or colours have been added. Organic food does not include foods that have been irradiated or Genetically Modified Organisms (GMOs).

Visit The Environmental Working Group website for consumer guides, www.ewg.org

Here are some nuggets:

- Avoid processed foods, trans fats, caffeine, and high fructose corn syrup. They are loaded with unhealthy carbs, artificial sweeteners, salt and preservatives.
- Food is either acid or alkaline (more correctly becomes alkaline or acid after the digestion):
  - ✓ Most fruits and vegetables are alkaline
  - ✓ Sugar, meat, and dairy are acidic

According to Lori Nichols Davies of the Holistic Cooking Academy "A meal should have a balance between the two types of food (at least two-third alkaline, one-third acidic. Fat has neutral pH)".

- Eat non-GMO (Genetically Modified Organism) produce and meats.
  - ✓ When it comes to produce, make a serious attempt to buy organic fruits and vegetables. Eat lots of fruits and vegetables (low in GI).
  - ✓ Buy eggs from free-run chicken (cage-free) farms.
  - ✓ Buy free-range poultry (chicken, turkey, etc.) raised on organic feeds.
  - ✓ Buy meat from grass fed animals.

✓ Buy wild fish rather than farmed fish.

- Choose vegetables that grow above the ground like cabbage, broccoli, cauliflower, and asparagus. Other low-glycemic vegetables that make healthy choices include mushrooms, green beans, leafy green vegetables, and tomatoes. Eat 3 to 5 servings of vegetables per day.

- Gluten is a special type of protein that is commonly found in rye, wheat, and barley. It is a major ingredient in most cereals and breads. If you are sensitive to gluten then avoid these grains.

- Avoid white foods (this is not a food term): Buy only whole grains, whole grain flours and brown rice. It is my contention that if we just avoid all white foods, it will decrease your risk factors for heart disease, diabetes and kidney problems by 25%. Imagine how much the government could save in health care costs!

  ✓ Potatoes (over 100 on the GI scale and over 20 on GL Index). Instead use sweet potato.

  ✓ White rice.

  ✓ Sugar: Ban white sugar. It is not food. It is a lethal toxin that creates killer fats and cancer. Replace a cup of sugar with a cup of Xylitol, or mix three-quarters of a teaspoon of stevia with a quarter cup of organic cane sugar. Sweeten porridge with molasses free of sulphites instead of white sugar.

  ✓ White flour (do not get misled by the "Enriched Flour" on the label). White wheat flour is bleached with chlorine gas.

  ✓ Commercial salt.

- Include protein, such as eggs, meats, fish, seeds and nuts, in all meals.

- Eat a savoury (non-sweet) breakfast, with protein and fat (almost like eating your lunch at your breakfast). Fat protects your teeth. Grains cause tooth decay.

- Healthy fat kills harmful bacteria that attack the gums. Seek adequate healthy fat such as organic butter or coconut oil. Saturated fats with vitamins A and D form strong cells in all tissues, especially the gums. Coconut oil and olive oil clean the liver; the liver keeps the blood clean; clean blood keeps the gums safe.

- Avoid all processed, boxed cereals (high in sugar).

- Make porridge in a double boiler.

- Avoid commercially baked goods and get into home baking.

- Eat oily fish, such as salmon or trout (they have high omega 3) twice a week.

- Add sea vegetables to soups and use dulse flakes in place of black pepper. We need about 60 trace minerals which are available from the sea.

- Eat lentils four times a week to increase your fibre to 10 grams per meal.

- There are 23 types of high fibre flours available today. Make pancakes with kamut, teff, quinoa or amaranth flours mixed with bean flours. Be adventurous with your diet.

- Live enzymes, vitamins, and minerals in foods are destroyed when cooked or fried. Explore some new ways of eating them:

  ✓ Eat all fruit and nuts raw.

  ✓ Eat some vegetables raw.

  ✓ Sprout some grains and soak nuts to make their dormant enzymes alive and to release their micronutrients.

Sprouting

Enzymes, vitamins and proteins in some plant foods are dormant or locked; this is nature's way of protecting them from unintended use or waste. As such, the nutrients in these foods are not readily absorbed by the body. However, you can enhance the availability of enzymes, proteins and vitamins in many legumes, grains and seeds by sprouting.

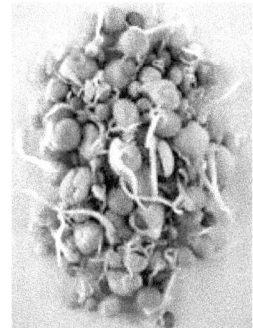

Resources http://sprouting.maxharoon.org

✓ Juice fruit and vegetables. Use a juicer with an augur or twin press (centrifugal juicers are not recommended due to their high RPM which destroys the nutrients).

According to Dr. Oksana Sawiak, DDS, "juice which is reconstituted from a concentrate is done so with tap water, which contains fluoride. That causes damage to the thyroid which then slows you down and makes you tired and fat."

Learn what to eat, what not to eat, how to eat, and when to eat.

Section 6:
Nutrition for Teeth
and Gum

Nutrition specific for the mouth is grouped as Food, Supplements and Herbs.

Food (Vegetables, Fruit, Nuts & Seeds)

A big factor in the health of the teeth is our entire body health. Even the best toothpaste or zealous brushing will not protect against decay if your diet is high in refined food, particularly refined sugar and flour which also increases the acidity.

Research in tooth health in people from various primitive cultures with healthy teeth (free from decay), revealed that their diet was much higher in vitamins and minerals, particularly calcium, magnesium, and vitamins A and D.

- **Rinse your mouth with water after eating anything.** Add a drop of essential oils (see Section 2 of Chapter 2) to the water. This special protocol before and after eating any food is essential to keep harmful bacteria from festering in your gums.

- **Eat food to enhance oral health.**

Live foods, such as fermented/lacto-fermented vegetables (sauerkraut, Kampucha) support the gut and feed the friendly bacteria. Eat yogurt, kefir or sour cream. Eat fermented foods daily. Buy sourdough bread. Avoid yeasted breads. Buy flatbread. Yeast feeds Candida and causes tooth decay. Japanese researchers have found that people taking two ounces of plain yogurt a day are less likely to have severe gum disease.

- **Salt kills harmful bacteria.**

Make sure it is quality salt with trace minerals (like Ocean Salt, Himalayan Salt). You can brush your teeth with salt and baking soda instead of toothpaste. Gargle with Himalayan pink crystal salt solution (made with water). This salt has 80+ minerals in colloidal form. It promotes tooth and bone health and is detoxifying.

- **Protect the enamel of your teeth.**

Acid and sugar are not good for your enamel. Phosphoric acid and sugar are significantly high ingredients in pop. They deplete calcium in bones and teeth. So does more than one cup of coffee (which is acidic). Instead choose water with lemon.

Vegetables

- Have something green every day, at every meal. The chlorophyll in the fresh green kills harmful bacteria. Bok choy, broccoli, cabbage, kale, lettuce, green peppers, spinach, wheatgrass are some of the green vegetables.
- Juice often: beet greens, celery, kale, carrots, peppers, and parsley.
- Use vegetable oils: hemp, flax-seed, coconut oil and evening Primrose.
- Munch on coconut and celery to fight gum disease.

Fruit

- Limit fruit to one to three servings per day. To sweeten homemade baked goods use apple juice. Malic acid in whole apples fights gum disease.

- A raw apple is known as Nature's Toothbrush. It helps remove plaque and provides vitamin C. Raw carrots supply vitamin A.

- Apricots, bananas, cranberries, figs, gooseberries, papaya and prunes are good choices in fruit.

- Cranberries and their juice (without sugar) stop cavity-causing bacteria from sticking to your teeth and prevent inflammatory gum disease.

Nuts, Grains & Seeds

- Almonds, brown Rice, flax-seed Oil, millet, sesame seeds, wheat bran/germ.

Nutritional Supplements & Herbs

The following dietary supplements are good for general and oral health:

- Minerals such as sodium, potassium, calcium, phosphorus, iron and magnesium.

- Chlorophyll is reported to help build enamel and prevent tooth decay. Vitamin C helps to reduce plaque build-up.

- Vitamins: A, B-complex, B-2, B-6, Bioflavonoids, Niacin, C, D3.

- Essential fatty acids, L-Glutathione, CoQ10, silica, zinc and Lactobacillus acidophilus.

- Chlorella, goldenseal (oral and local), lobelia, myrrh, oatstraw, sage tea, skullcap, tea tree oil (topical use only).

- Valerian Root.

Vitamin A and C are needed for the absorption of calcium, and calcium is an essential element in our teeth. Sea vegetables are rich in calcium and most green plants have significant amounts of chlorophyll, phosphorus, vitamins A and C, all of which are needed for calcium absorption. `

Section 7:
Last Word

You just finished reading a lot of strategies for living a healthy holistic life. It may be overwhelming to grasp and apply all of these techniques, so start with a handful after evaluating your preferences and convictions.

A summary of some of the tips given throughout the book:

Remember, health is priceless. Without it, life is no fun. Health is Wealth

- Keep your oral hygiene efforts at a high level.
- Use natural products like essential oils, herbs and homeopathic remedies to protect yourself and kill infections.
- Avoid toxic exposures from products like commercial toothpastes and mouthwashes.
- Nourish yourself with clean, organic, live food.
- Take supplemental vitamins and minerals.
- Get plenty of fresh air and exercise to oxygenate your body (infections do not like oxygen, outdoor air has more oxygen than indoor air).
- Keep the pH of your body on the slightly alkaline side to reduce inflammation.
- Learn stress-fighting techniques like meditation or yoga to keep your immune system strong.
- Find a biologic dentist. Make sure that he/she does much more than simply "biologic protocol to remove the mercury amalgam".
- Find a physician who knows Orthomolecular or Functional Medicine or consult a naturopath or a knowledgeable Wellness Consultant.
- Drink clean non-chlorinated, fluoride-free water.
- Question and research every invasive procedure offered – be it medical or dental.
- Avoid drugs to the best of your ability and question or research every prescription diligently.

APPENDICES

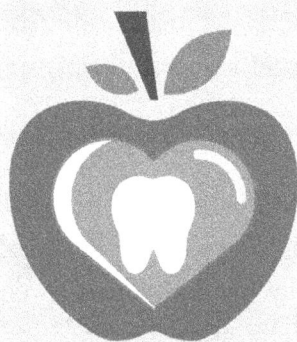

All resources mentioned in the
Appendices are provided as
clickable links on the book's website
under RESOURCES.

A. FAQ (Frequently Asked Questions)

Q 1: Can you brush your teeth too much?

Yes, if you brush with a hard and with a stiff brush, with too much force, or too often, you can wear away the delicate gum tissues and cause a recession. If you use a back and forth sawing motion of your brush, you can even abrade the enamel – the hardest tissue in our body.

Q 2: Can you get away with not using toothpaste?

If there is no infection in your mouth, you need no toothpaste. If there is an infection, you can use disinfecting or herbal product like Aloe Vera or an essential oil product like, oil of oregano or tea tree oil to kill the germs. You can also use an Ionic toothbrush, which produces negative ions that kill bacteria.

Q 3: Can you get away with not using any mouthwash?

Most people need no mouthwash to make their breath fresh (if they have no infections). However to kill infection or prevent germs a non-toxic herbal mouthwash can be a good addition to your oral hygiene kit.

Q 4: Is it better to brush immediately after a meal? Does it apply to all kinds of meals?

The best time to brush is immediately after eating. The more sticky or sweet the food is, the more important is the urgency of brushing. Cheese and apples are known to have a natural cleansing action.

Q 5: Is it better to wait to brush after eating fruits or fruit juices?

Many fruits are very high in sugar and/or acid and will harm the teeth, especially when taken as juice where there is no mechanical cleaning action of the fibrous part of the fruit. When brushing is not convenient, like after lunch at work, it is better to avoid sweet fruits and juices.

First rinse with salt water/mouthwash, then wait for 20 minutes before brushing your teeth.

Q 6: Do I have to brush after every meal?

It is more important to avoid the germs getting into your mouth than obsessing about the brushing. I recommend a routine of brushing after breakfast, and a complete regimen of 7 Steps after supper (last meal before bed). This is adequate to prevent most food related decay.

Q 7: I know Mercury Amalgams are not good but how can I live with them; I am too scared to get them out of my teeth?

It is only safe to have them removed by a biologically trained dentist. Otherwise, develop a comprehensive and regular heavy metal detox program with your Wellness Counsellor; avoid very hot or acidic foods, do not have your fillings polished by the hygienist and do not chew gum.

Q 8: Can I live with my root canal?

You may get away with the low-grade infection and the toxins it produces for many years, but be aware that root canals are not healthy in 75% of the cases. It can be a factor in many diseases especially if the body is already under the stress of emotional trauma, viral attack or severe weather. It may not cause a problem today, but it can add to your pile of 'sins'.

Q. 9: Why do I hear that root canals are not a good idea?

Embalming a dead tooth causes infection and toxins to be released into the body constantly (to some degree) as long as the tooth is there. Research by Dr. Weston Price, Dr. Rosenow and Dr. Haley showed that most root canal treated teeth are not safe for your immune system. *Suffice it to say that in the thirty years that I was practicing biological dentistry, there was not one case of breast cancer that did not have a root canal, infection or toxic restoration on a tooth on the breast meridian on the same side as the cancer.*

Q 10: If I am practising doing do-it-yourself scaling after every meal, as described in this book, do I have to visit a dental hygienist?

If there is no calculus, stain or plaque, and your gums are tight and light pink with no pockets, there is no need to see your dentist or hygienist for cleanings. It is wise to have yourself checked at least once a year, and to follow up with a professional cleaning if necessary. I encourage you to get a microscopic imaging of your plaque done before you request a cleaning, especially if you have had challenges with gum disease.

Q 11: Where do the acids that cause tooth decay come from?

Bacteria feed on sugar and carbohydrates that we eat. The end product they produce is acid.

Q 12: How is tooth decay formed? What is the process?

The acid formed by the bacteria digesting the sugar etches and dissolves enamel. Once the enamel is penetrated, there is a softer and more vulnerable layer underneath called dentin. Like bone, dentin is comprised of tubules that carry bacteria deep into the tooth and cause cavities to mushroom rapidly.

Q 13: Tooth Sealants - are they good at stopping tooth decay?

Research has shown that sealants can seal in decay and often lift at the edges, and that can cause more decay than it prevents. However if the grooves in your teeth are very deep, properly done sealants are a good idea.

Q 14: Can you reuse dental floss after washing in running hot water?

You could sterilize floss by running boiling water or peroxide on it, but you have to consider the time and effort it takes vs. the cost of a new piece.

Q 15: Can you catch gum disease from other people?

Most definitely! Gum disease is contagious.

Q 16: Is gum disease hereditary?

Gum disease, like any infection is not hereditary but we are vulnerable to infections from our loved ones by the act of kissing if the loved one has a gum disease.

Q 17: Is Acidity in the mouth the same throughout the day and night?

During the night when we sleep our saliva stops flowing. This changes the pH of our saliva, as can medications, certain food, tiredness and stress.

Q 18: Will gargling with salt water immediately after the meal help if I am unable to brush immediately?

A saturated mixture of salt and water will kill germs very effectively and prevent infections as well as decay.

Q 19: Is there a minimum amount of time required for brushing to achieve a well-done job?

It usually takes a minimum of 4 minutes to do a good job on a mouthful of teeth.

Q 20: How often should one clean the toothbrush, rubber stimulator or tongue scraper? Can you use soap for cleaning or do you have to use some kind of the sterilization process?

Toothbrushes, rubber stimulators and tongue scrapers can be cleaned daily with ethyl alcohol, hydrogen peroxide, colloidal silver or even boiling water. The more infected the person is, the more often they need to sterilize their oral hygiene tools. If a person has a mouth clear of germs and parasites, it is probably enough to sterilize oral care instruments once a month as long as they are kept in a clean environment in between uses.

Q 21: Is it OK to brush your teeth immediately after eating an acidic fruit, like lemon or pineapple? Does the acid in the fruit make the teeth or enamel softer?

If you hold the fruit with your teeth or keep it in your mouth for a long time, it will affect the enamel. If you chew and swallow in the normal way, you can clean them or rinse with alkaline water immediately to reduce acidity before the saliva has a chance to buffer the acid by itself. We are in a constant process of decalcification and recalcification of our teeth. When decalcification is faster, you get decay, when recalcification outstrips decalcification, decay is prevented, and there are no cavities.

Q 22: The enamel-protecting toothpastes, do they work? What about the claim of Remineralisation?

The enamel-protecting or recalcifying toothpaste uses Calcium to recalcify enamel that has been decalcified and yes, they do work over a long period of time. They are much better than the desensitizing toothpastes (toothpastes for sensitive teeth) that use fluoride. Some new toothpastes containing Nano-Hydroxyapatite do a good job of Remineralisation of teeth. Hydroxyapatite is the main component of enamel that gives the tooth a bright white appearance.

Q 23: What is the difference between bacteria, a virus and a pathogen?

All of them are micro-organisms/germs. See Glossary for their descriptions.

Many human illnesses are caused by pathogenic (disease-causing) bacteria or viruses. Bacterial infections can be treated successfully with antibiotics, but antibiotics are useless against viral infections.

Q 24: How do I protect my children from all the sugar around them in school, at birthday parties and Halloween?

If refined sugar were introduced now as a new food or chemical, it would never pass FDA/Health Canada approval because it causes tooth decay, diabetes, heart disease and obesity and is addicting immediately upon first taste. Yes, until the child tastes sugar, they do not crave it. With sugar found in all kinds of unsuspected products, the best advice is: Allow the child whatever the sugar product they want BUT ONLY once a day e.g. after supper. This reduces the exposure of the teeth to ONE acid attack a day and reduces decay incidence. It also eventually reduces the total amount of sugar ingested by becoming self-limiting because of how much a child will take at one time.

Q. 25: My mother lost her teeth to gum disease at 42 so will I as well?

Only if you share the same infections and do not get rid of them. Get a microscopic analysis of the plaque so you can identify and fight the enemy.

Q. 26: I grind my teeth. What causes that?

Here, are some causes and some solutions:

- Stress: Walking outside, self-hypnosis, Homeopathy and herbal treatments.
- Parasites: Do a proper herbal cleanse.
- Uneven bite muscle imbalance: Consider bite plates and orthodontics.
- Spinal misalignment: Visit a Chiropractor

If grinding and clenching is associated with sleep apnea, then the person is trying to open his or her airways. The tongue falls back into the throat, blocking the airway breathing momentarily blocks.

Q. 27: I have a toothache but the dentist cannot find anything wrong.

Some possible causes:

- It could be that the bite is high – for instance on a new filling or after orthodontics.
- That the amalgam filling in the tooth has expanded and cracked the tooth.
- It could be a blockage on the meridian of that tooth causing a toothache.

All these situations are invisible and hard to diagnose. X-rays do not readily show cracks in the tooth or the blockage of a meridian.

Q. 28: What causes white spots on my teeth?

It is called Fluorosis and is caused by too much ingested fluoride. It also occurs in bones and organs.

Q. 29: Is fluoride not good for teeth?

Studies show fluoridated water does nothing except poison our thyroids, make our bones brittle and cause us to become dumber. It also causes cancers. There is some evidence that topical fluoride may have some benefit, but I would not use it on my kids.

Q. 30: I heard eating an apple, or some hard cheese at the end of a meal has some benefit. How does that work?

It helps reduce cavities, scrubs teeth and increases alkalinity.

Q. 31: Is toothpaste necessary to clean teeth properly?

Most toothpaste brands are toxic; the foaming agent in toothpastes (SLS), isopropyl alcohol, sweeteners are toxic. Many toothpastes coat plaque rather than removing it and often irritate the gums. Toothpastes that have only herbs and essential oils will kill pathogens and clean teeth much better and more safely. The best toothpaste I am aware of is sold only through holistic dental offices, wellness practitioners and health food stores.

Q. 32: Are mouthwashes good to use?

Most have alcohol as an ingredient that burns gums and causes gum disease rather than curing it. Some even have sugar or aspartame. Use a mouthwash with essential oils and herbs or make one as suggested in the Chapter 2 (Section 7) of the book.

Q. 33: What is your opinion about implants?

Implants are the most elegant and conservative way of replacing a missing tooth. The only problem is that they are metal (titanium). Some have been shown to be polluted with nickel. I hope that zirconium implants will take their place soon to make it safe for the body. Zirconium has been used successfully in Europe for over twenty years and is being widely used in the U.S.A.

Q. 34: Is there anything wrong with having braces?

Most orthodontics done today involve metal brackets and wires. There are nickel-free brackets but as of yet no nickel free wires, so detoxing the body actively from the nickel during treatment would be a good idea.

Invisalign and Occlus-O-Guide, are brace alternative appliances made of vinyl or clear plastic (no metal). These are worth exploring.

Q. 35: Since I got my last crown, I have a burning feeling on my tongue. What is causing it?

It could be electro galvanic current between the crown and another metal in your mouth like a mercury amalgam filling, implant, or metal-based denture. Alternatively, the crown could contain palladium, which can cause severe neurological symptoms including burning tongue.

Q. 36: I nurse my baby. Why does my baby have cavities on her front teeth?

Baby bottle Caries are caused by the baby falling asleep with the bottle in her mouth causing the milk to pool around the teeth. The sugar in the milk rots the teeth. If the mother and baby fall asleep while nursing, the same thing happens. Always take the bottle or breast out of the baby's mouth before the baby falls asleep. The only thing in the bottle of a sleeping baby should be water.

B. Useful Websites

Website Resources are given throughout the book to make them more relevant and contextual. Some additional resources are given below.

worldfitness.com/

www.perfectbalancetherapies.com

www.toxicteeth.org

www.hugginsappliedhealing.com/

www.naturallifemagazine.com/9702/mercury.htm

www.shirleys-wellness-cafe.com

www.simplyteeth.com/

www.nidcr.nih.gov/OralHealth/Topics/ToothDecay/

http://www.holisticmed.com/dental/

Find a Mercury Free & Mercury Safe Dentist page on Dr. McGuire's web sites www.dentalwellness4u.com and www.mercuryfreenow.com.

Chemical Free Body Care, Biomedical, etc.

stason.org/articles/wellbeing/health/Chemical-Free-Bodycare.html

Hidden dangers lurking in your cosmetics and personal care products

www.energygrid.com/health/2006/11kf-personalcare.html

The Center for the Disease Control: Part of Department of Health and Human Services, USA Government

www.cdc.gov/search.do?q=mercury+amalgam&spell=1&ie=utf8

The **Agency for Toxic Substances and Disease Registry (ATSDR), USA**

www.atsdr.cdc.gov/phs/phs.asp?id=112&tid=24

Bernard Windham, Chemical Engineer, 52 pages Report with 527 Citations

www.flcv.com/amalg6.html

List of websites of medical studies and the USA Government Agencies www.flcv.com/indexa.html

A professional source of information on biomedical topics is PubMed, www.ncbi.nlm.nih.gov/pubmed/ PubMed was developed by the National Center for Biotechnology Information (NCBI), www.ncbi. nlm.nih.gov/ at the National Library of Medicine (NLM) www.nlm.nih. gov/, located at the National Institutes of Health (NIH) www.nih.gov/ It was developed in conjunction with publishers of biomedical literature as a search tool for accessing literature citations and linking to full-text journals at websites of participating publishers.

The Society for Science-Based Medicine (SfSBM.org): a community for like-minded individuals, both in and out of health care, who support the goals of Science-Based Medicine. This website was created to promote and discuss our views — the SfSBM is the next step towards educating consumers, professionals, and legislators. Also http://www. sciencebasedmedicine.org

C. Holistic Dental Organizations

Holistic Dental Hygiene practice

The licence to practice dental hygiene is called R.D.H (Registered Dental Hygienist).

The following websites provide more information about tools, software and products used by the hygienist (more are posted on the book website):

The Eco-Dentistry Association provides Education, Standards & Connection to support the success of our industry and the wellness lifestyle of the patients we serve. www.ecodentistry.org/

Dental Clearance Center directory www.dentalclearancecenters.com

Holistic Dental Organizations

D.D.S. refers to the academic degree of Doctor of Dental Surgery for the dentist. Some universities are also offering Doctor of Dental Medicine (D.M.D).

Since 1978, the **Holistic Dental Association** has provided support and guidance to practitioners of holistic and alternative dentistry, as well as informing the public of the benefits of holistic dentistry for their health and well-being. www.holisticdental.org/

The American Academy for Oral Systemic Health (AAOSH) is an organization of health care leaders and health professionals dedicated to the relationship of oral health and whole body health. Its vision is to improve inter- disciplinary healthcare and collaboration, and the health of people everywhere by changing public and professional awareness of the mouth-body health links. This group has memberships from both mainstream and holistic dentists. www.aaosh.org/

International Academy of Oral Medicine & Toxicology (IAOMT) is the Vanguard of Science - Based Biological Dentistry. The IAOMT is a network of dental, medical and research professionals who seek to raise the standards of scientific biocompatibility in the dental practice with information from the latest interdisciplinary research. iaomt.org/

The International Academy of Biological Dentistry and Medicine (IABDM), iabdm.org/

D. Dangers of Dental Mercury - Resources

The International Academy of Oral Medicine and Toxicology Amalgam Video, www.youtube.com/watch?v=GgXsCixF6Qs

Campaign for Mercury-Free Dentistry, www.toxicteeth.org/

Mercury Policy Project, mercurypolicy.org/

Mercuriados, www.mercuriados.org/ (Spain)

Dental Amalgam Mercury Solutions (DAMS) at www.amalgam.org is a patient support organization for people with chronic mercury conditions.

Videos: www.toxicteeth.org/dental-mercury-videos.aspx

Safety of Dental Amalgam, Health Canada position:

www.hc-sc.gc.ca/dhp-mps/pubs/md-im/dent_amalgam-eng.php

Dr. Tom McGuire www.mercuryfreenow.com/tom/tomart.html

Dental Wellness Institute www.dentalwellness4u.com

The Mercury Papers - The Most Expensive Medical Mistake in the History of the World

www.positivehealth.com/issue/issue-178-january-2011 www.wholisticresearch.com/info/artshow.php3?artid=20

Natural Life Magazine, January/February 1997 issue with the title: "Mercury Fillings: A Time Bomb in Your Head" by Charles W. Moore, www.naturallifemagazine.com/9702/mercury.htm

Watch a dramatic video of mercury vapour gassing out from an amalgam dental filling that has outraged the world iaomt.org/videos/

Also, research for David Kennedy, DDS on www.youtube.com

Royal College of Dental Surgeons of Ontario, search for Policy Statement on amalgam fillings www.rcdso.org

E. Books About Dental Health

Brushing Well, Helen Frost

Food for Your Healthy teeth, Helen Frost

Good Teeth from Birth to Death, Dr. Gerard F. Judd, Ph.D.

Healthy Teeth, Healthy Body, Dr. Tom McGuire

Healthy Teeth & Gums, Edward Miller

Healthy Teeth, Dr. Marvin J. Schissel, Dr. John Dodes

It's all in Your Head, the link between mercury amalgam and illness, Dr. Hal A. Huggins

Mercury Detoxification: The Natural Way to Remove Mercury from Your Body, Dr. Tom McGuire

Mercury Fillings: A Time Bomb in Your Head, Charles W. Moore. The Natural Life Magazine, Jan. /Feb. 1997,

Take Care of Your Teeth, Don L. Curry

The Root Canal Cover-Up by Dr. George Meinig

Dr. Weston Price wrote over 1100 pages of studies about root canals, some of which is contained in this book. George Meinig was one of the 10 founders of the Association of Endodontics and a dentist who performed thousands of root canals over his long career. It wasn't until his retirement that he took the time to read Dr. Price's work from the 1920's and was shocked at the pertinent information and quality studies that had been withheld from public knowledge. "A woman with breast cancer is worth between $800,000 and $1.2 million to the American Medical Association system". A woman with healthy breast makes no one any money!

"Quote from "Breast Health Exposed".

The Tooth Trip, Dr. Tom McGuire

The Poison In Your Teeth, Dr. Tom McGuire

The Tooth Book, Edward Miller

Tooth Truth, Dr. Frank Jerome

Toxic Dentistry Exposed: The Link Between Dentistry and Chronic Disease, Dr. Graeme Munro-Hall BDS and Dr. Lilian Munro-Hall BDS

Your Toxic Teeth: A guide to Mercury Poisoning from Dental Fillings, Dr. Murray J. Vimy, DMD

Your Mouth: The Gateway to a Healthier You, Dana G. Colson

More than two hundred books, under various categories, about Health, Pharmaceutical System, Medicine Business, Food, exploitation of health, etc. are listed at

life-transformation-institute.org/resources/books/index.htm

Books about Pharmaceutical System and environmental health are listed at

life-transformation-institute.org/resources/books/environment_
health_books.htm

Books Recommended by Dr. Al Sears, MD

life-transformation-institute.org/resources/books/dr_sears_
recommendations.htm

Books about Macrobiotics

life-transformation-institute.org/resources/books/macrobiotics_books.
htm

F. Life Transformation Institute (LTI)

*"Everyone thinks of changing the world but
no one thinks of changing himself"*
LEO TOLSTOY

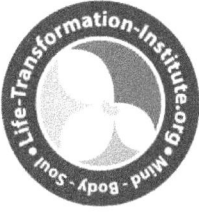

We spend our lifetime taking care of others; and in the process, we neglect to look after ourselves. If this message resonates with you, then join us in a sojourn to take charge of yourself - through self-management of your mind, body and spirit.

The Life Transformation Institute (LTI) is a not-for-profit community group of collaborative kindred spirits who empower life by sharing their cumulative knowledge and wisdom to raise awareness in the body, mind and spirit.

LTI achieves its objectives by:

- Networking events/lunches with practitioners
- Presentations and Workshops
- Resource Intensive Website life-transformation-institute.org/
- Publications of Articles, books and online videos

We have conducted many meetings, talks and workshops, since 2008. You can review photos and reports of these events at:

life-transformation-institute.org/events

Join **Facebook group https://www.facebook.com/groups/ LTinstitute/**

G. Credits

We acknowledge the following sources of information. The acknowledgment is not necessarily an endorsement of their products, services or the contents on their website:

Trans4mind - "Minds, like parachutes, function better when open" www.trans4mind.com

Wikipedia - en.wikipedia.org/wiki/Sprouting

Dental health questions dentistry.about.com/od/dentalhealth/l/bldosanddonts.htm

Stats in Chapter 1: National Institute of Dental and Craniofacial Research

www.nidcr.nih.gov/DataStatistics/

... Many more references and resources mentioned throughout the book

Credits for Images

Juliusz Gajus for profile photo www.juliuszgajus.com

Structure of a Tooth www.studiodentaire.com/

Formulation of acid The Health Age www.thehealthage.com

UK Tooth Charts www.dentalfearcentral.org/resources/tooth-charts

Various images http://dreamstime.com

H. Authors and Our Medical Team

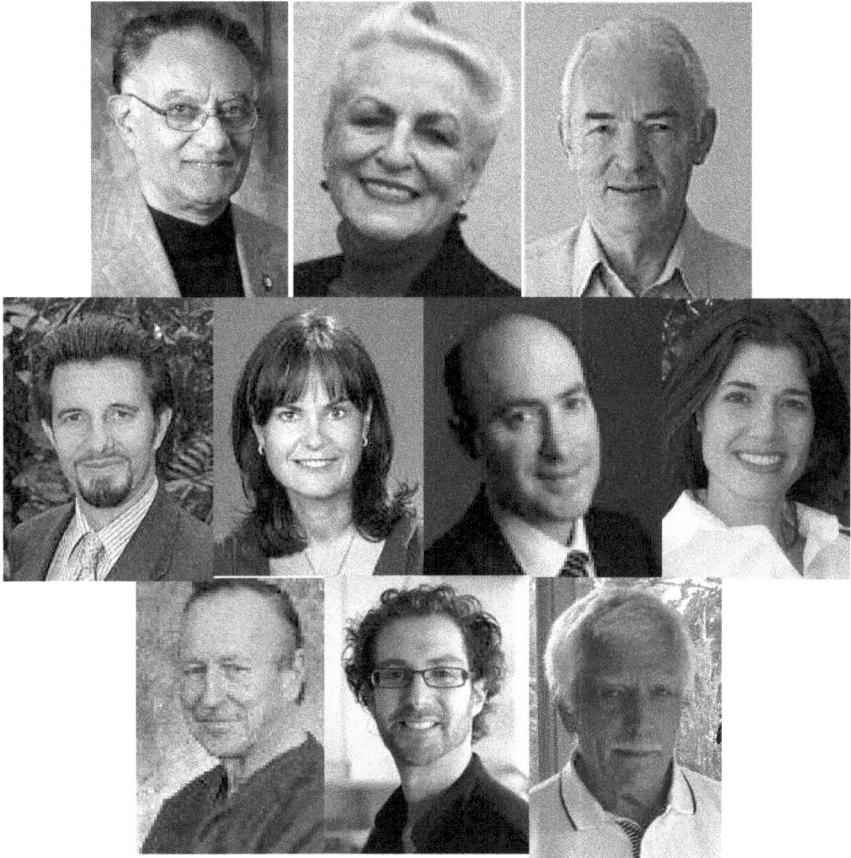

From left to right:

Row 1: Authors: Max Haroon, Dr. Oksana Sawiak and Klaus Ferlow
Row 2: Contributors: Dr. Brian Clement, Dr. Dana Colson, Dr. Eric Grief, and Dr. Iris Kivity-Chandler
Row 3: Contributors: Dr. Brian McLean, Dr. Michael Schecter and Dr. Hans-Jurgen Schwartz

Max Haroon, a social entrepreneur and an author is a retired e-Marketing specialist, who always has been interested in holistic health and alternative medicine. He is the founder of the Society of Internet Professionals, www.

sipgroup.org and Life Transformation Institute www.life-transformation-institute.org

Max has authored seven books in the Life Learning Series, in conjunction with subject matter experts. The books are based on his life lessons learned in a heuristic way. He has architected many websites and digital publications. Review his publications and postings at www.maxharoon.org email: max@maxharoon.org

Dr. Oksana M. Sawiak, DDS, IMD, MAGD, AIAOMT, **Integrative Wellness Consultant.** Dr. Sawiak practiced clinical family dentistry from 1966-2008 focusing on mercury-free/biological dentistry. She lectures in holistic dentistry, non-surgical gum treatment, pain control, hypnosis, practice management, temporo-mandibular joint pain and dysfunction, and detoxification. Dr. Sawiak is the past Vice President of the International Academy of Oral Medicine and Toxicology. www.drsawiak.com/. Contact (905)279-6619, drsawiak@drsawiak.com

Klaus Ferlow, HMH, HA, is an author, innovator, lecturer, researcher, founder, co-owner of Ferlow Botanicals, www.ferlowbotanicals.com, Vancouver, B.C., which is a company he founded in 1975. Klaus is an Honorary Master Herbalist Dominion Herbal College and a Board member of the Health Action Network Society, Professional Herbal Advocate (HA) of the Canadian Herbalist's Association of B.C., and belongs to a number of health organizations. Contact (604) 820-1777, klausferlow1@gmail.com

CONTRIBUTORS (alphabetically)

Dr. Brain R. Clement, Brian Clement, Ph.D., L.N. Director, Hippocrates Health Institute, (USA) has spent more four decades studying nutrition and natural health care. Brian has conducted educational programs in more than 25 countries around the globe and is the author of numerous books including his recent best-selling book, *Living Foods for Optimum Health* http://www.hippocratesinst.org/

Dr. Dana Colson brings together leading-edge technology and natural medicine to give clients award-winning smiles that enhance their lives. Dana is an author and has lectured internationally. Contact (416) 482-2133 or www.allsmiles.ca

Dr. Eric M. Grief, M.D. is a staff physician at The Bramalea Health Center and medical director for an international weight-loss company centred in Toronto, Canada. His research interests include preventive medicine, family counselling and nutrition education. He offers communication improvement seminars and has authored "Get Diagnosed Fast". Contact: egrief@aol.com

Dr. Iris Kivity-Chandler, DDS, Cert. Ortho, M. Sc. Toronto, Orthodontics, TMD, Craniofacial pain, Headaches and Sleep Disordered Breathing. Science is discovering more and more connections between the health of our jaws and mouth and our overall health. Iris practices in Toronto and Thornhill clinics. www.kivitychandlerorthotmd.com. Contact: (416) 787-9060

Dr. Brian D. McLean graduated from the University of Toronto dental school in 1969. Brian has practiced general dentistry in Mississauga, Barrie and Toronto since 1970. During that time, he has discovered that the dogma which drives the health sciences often conflicts with the scientific method. He often refers to himself as a "recovering dentist".

Dr. Michael Schecter, keeps current by attending Biological Dental lectures and workshops and through his membership in The International Academy of Oral Medicine and Toxicology (IAOMT), conversely he also give talks along with other practitioners to educate them. Contact 416 665 1145 or www.schecterdental.com

Dr. Hans-Jurgen Schwartz has devoted his dental career to practicing healthy, holistic, non-invasive, biocompatible dentistry. He is also a proponent of making the dental office occupationally safe regarding mercury and he strives to protect the patient, the staff, and the environment from excessive and unnecessary exposure to mercury at the dental office. Contact: (905) 294-8668 or hans@holisticdentalhealth.ca

I. Acknowledgments

*Something that has always puzzled me all my life is why, when
I am in special need of help, the good deed is usually done by
somebody on whom I have no claim.*

~William Feather

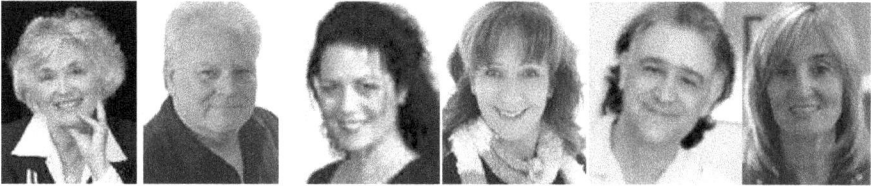

L-R: Lori Nichols Davies, Vaughn Dragland, Victoria DaCosta, Lesley Ann Marcovich, Dr. Ebi Taebi, Sharon Walsh

A giant thanks to all who have reviewed this book and were brave enough to provide me with their valuable comments. All reviews are posted on the book's website.

Book Writing (and all other tasks related to it), along with the design of the website are particularly demanding and challenging tasks, and credit of the book in your hand goes to the following members of the multidiscipline book team:

- Andrea Chambers, editor for printed words for an initial edit.
- Geoff Fridd for editing the language Usage.
- Lesley Ann Marcovich, author "The Biography Workbook" for editing the book.
- Lori Nichols Davies, holistic nutritional consultant for nutritional review.
- Muhammad Mollah, Webmaster for designing the book's interactive website.
- Nerissa Thomson for designing the logo of the Life Transformation Institute.

- Phil Feilds, health educator with background in biochemistry and cellular biology.

- Sharon Walsh for her expertise in use of essential oils for oral health and conditions.

- Vaughn Dragland, Eclipse Technologies Inc. for book covers and layout design.

- Victoria DaCosta, RDH, BSDH, SHC, a Systemic Hygiene Consultant for review and contributions.

I am greatly indebted to all my co-authors, medical team and other practitioners for their contributions. The book will not have the credibility and technical content without their insights.

J. Study Guides

Learning from Classic Books to Transform You

Some books have shifted the paradigm of societies, yet some of us have not read them because we are unaware of it, do not have time to read or they are difficult to comprehend. These guides, called "Study Guides" will provide key insights from the book and a few will have a full text and audio recordings.

Study Guides provides:

- ▶ Synopsis of the book and its Author
- ▶ What Others Say About the Book
- ▶ Quotes from the Book
- ▶ Key Insights from the Book
- ▶ Discussion Points
- ▶ Resources for further explorations of the book
- ▶ Resources for Mind, Body and Soul Studies

The Life Transformation Institute (LTI) has embarked on publishing the following Seven Study Guides. They will be available for a small donation of $5 for each book.

- As the Man Thinketh by James Allen
- The Prophet by Kahlil Gibran
- Secrets of the Millionaire Mind by Harv Ecker
- Thoughts Are Things by Prentice Mulford
- Molecules of Emotion by Dr. Candace Pert
- The Brain That Changes Itself by Norman Doidge
- Living Enlightenment by Andrew Cohen
- Blink by Malcolm Gladwell

Details http://tiny.cc/bookguides

An education project of The Life Transformation Institute (LTI), a not-for-profit, empowering life by sharing wisdom.

K. Educational Presentations

Our authors are available to give talks and presentations on various aspects of mind, body, soul and more. We will appreciate such opportunities from community groups and organizations.

Dental Health

1.   Seven Steps to Holistic Dental Health

2.   How Toxic Are You? Toxicity from Your Body Care Products

3.   Systemic Diseases Connections: Chronic Medical Conditions Linked to Your Dental Health

4.   Dental Conditions and Mercury Fillings

5.   Self-Assessment of Your Dental Health and Dental Office

6.   Oil Pulling and Other Oral Health Therapies

7.   Nutrition for Your Dental and Overall Health

Miscellaneous

1.   Seven Steps to Manage Your Stress: Is There a Switch to Turn off Your Stress?

2.   Food According to Various Traditions and Nutrition: Seven Principles of Nutrition.

3.   Seven Essentials to Make Your Food Alive: Enhance the Availability of Dormant Enzymes of Plant Based Food.

4.   Seven-Steps to Re-Boot Your Body: A Holistic Guide for Well-being of Your Mind, Body and Soul.

5.   A Seven-Step Strategy for Your Career Success: A Guide for Job Seekers and Entrepreneurs.

For further information, please contact:

Max Haroon | Founder | Life Transformation Institute

416-891-4937 or by email book@7stepsdentalhealth.com

L. Publications by the Life Transformation Institute

Life Learning Series
Books on various aspects of Life and Living

1. Seven-Imperatives to Healthy Aging: A Holistic Guide for Well-being of Your Mind, Body and Soul for All Ages

2. A Seven Step Strategy for Your Career Success

   - Guide to Successful Professionalism and Employment

3. 7 Steps to Dental Health (this book)

   - A Holistic Guide to a Healthy Mouth and Body

4. Seven Essentials to Make Your Food Alive

   - Enhance the Availability of Dormant Enzymes of Plant Based Food.

5. *Sprouting and Fermenting to Unlock Nutrition*

   - 7 Ways to Enhance the Availability of Dormant Enzymes of Plant Based Food

6. Seven-Steps to Publish Your Book

   - Guide to Write, Publish and Market Your Book in All Media

7. Seven Steps to Reboot Your Well Being: Why Do You Get Sick and How Can You Heal*

Articles

   - Weight Management and Metabolism
   - Create Your Own Miracles - Manifest Whatever You want
   - Why You Should Write Your Life Story
   - Significance of Website Linkages
   - Human Beings are Resilient
   - 100 Inspirational Books

Book Discussion Kits

- The Prophet by Kahlil Gibran
- As the Man Thinketh by James Allen
- Secrets of the Millionaire Mind by Harv Ecker

Videos

- Why Should You Write Your Life Story
- Planning for End of Life Care

http://maxharoon.org/ and http://life-transformation-institute.org/

7 Steps to Dental Health:
A Holistic Guide to a Healthy Mouth and Body is available
in the following formats

	Format	Source	URL	ISBN	Price
1	Paperback	Amazon Store	http://www.amazon.com/dp/0987882805	978-0987882806	$22.50
2	Paperback	Create Space Store	https://www.createspace.com/4421931	978-0987882806	$22.50
3	Paperback	Book's Website	http://7stepsdentalhealth.com/?page_id=2 The price includes an e-Book on Sprouting & Fermentation and shipping.	978-0987882806	Cdn $25.00
4	eReader	Kindle Online Store	http://www.amazon.com/dp/B00GXS7D8A	978-0987882820	$9.41
5	eReader	KOBO online store	http://store.kobobooks.com/en-CA/ebook/7-steps-to-dental-health	978-0987882820	$10.41
6	Digital Book	Book's Website	http://7stepsdentalhealth.com/?page_id=2 The price includes an e-Book on Sprouting & Fermentation and shipping.	978-0987882813	Cdn $15.00
7	Colour Paperback	Create Space Store	https://www.createspace.com/4767492	978-1499204025	$39.00

All prices are in US $ except where specified.

Hydroponic Sprout Grower
Grow Your Own Organic Source of Enzymes and Vitamins

Enzymes, vitamins and proteins in some plant foods are dormant or locked when you eat them. You can enhance the availability of these nutrients by sprouting seeds, grains and legumes. A sprouts are live plant (root, leaves and stem) when eating them.

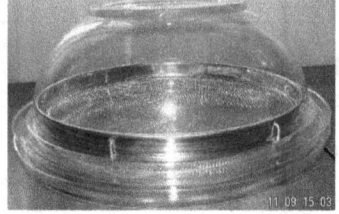

Tony Hornick's sprouter is by far the best designed sprouter available today.

What is Special

This sprouter is guaranteed to bring you years and years of fresh, delicious and nutritious sprouts for you and your family!

- The grains/beans/seeds rest on the mesh tray just above the water, **eliminating mould**. (Sprouting in glass jars by submerging grains/beans in the water, increases their susceptibility to mould).

- The dome also maintains humidity to provide the right environment for propagation.

- Being plastic it is light weight which allows any gases to escape and fresh air to go in.

- The plastic is food grade and free from BPA and other plastic toxicity.

- Hard cardboard gift box

Natural source of ALL nutrients to keep YOU healthy (a natural multi-vitamin and mineral pill at fraction of the cost)

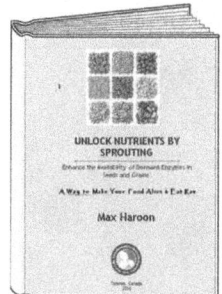

Your Investment

$35 includes a "Sprouting Seeds and Grains to Unlock Nutrients" *http://sprouting.maxharoon.org/ to purchase and download resources*

Max Haroon | guide@life-transformation-institute.org

All proceed are donated to Life Transformation Institute, a non-profit, to propagate holistic education

SPROUTING SEEDS AND GRAINS TO UNLOCK NUTRIENTS

Grow Your Own Organic Source of Enzymes and Vitamins

Make Your Food Alive & Eat Raw

This book was written after researching the claim "Grow Your Own Organic Source of Enzymes and Vitamins". Yes, sprouting is powerful method to make food alive. Various sprouting methods were explored with various seeds and grains.

- Seven Ways to Make Your Food Alive
- Sprouting Seeds and Grains
- Benefits of Sprouting
- How to Sprout
- Soaking time and Nutrients of various Seeds and Grains
- Eating and Drinking Alkaline Foods
- Principles of Nutrition

Your Investment

$10 Purchase your eBook at

http://sprouting.maxharoon.org/

Max Haroon | guide@life-transformation-institute.org

All proceed are donated to Life Transformation Institute, a non-profit, to propagate holistic education

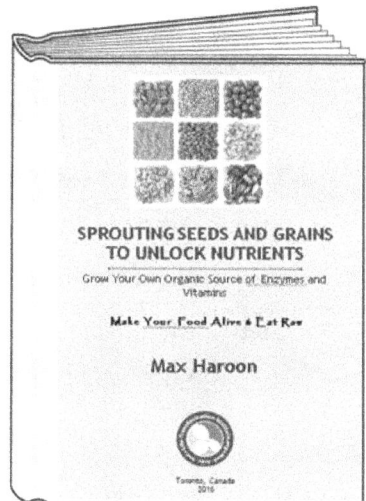

A Seven-Step Strategy for Your Career Success

A Professional Guide for Job Seekers and Entrepreneurs

This book is based on the Author's presentations at various career conferences and job fairs. Max Haroon has been on both sides of the fence, one as an employers and another as employee, which has helped to write this short guide.

He has devised a seven-step strategy for success that you can apply to many situations in your life, which could be job searching, all other aspects of your career or in a business as an entrepreneur.

Step 1: Establishing Credibility

Step 2: Business Networking

Step 3: Attitude & Acculturation

Step 4: Volunteering

Step 5: Mentoring & Coaching

Step 6: Life Long Learning

Step 7: Holistic Life and Living

Tips and techniques outlined below will help you whether you are in a native environment or a foreign one.

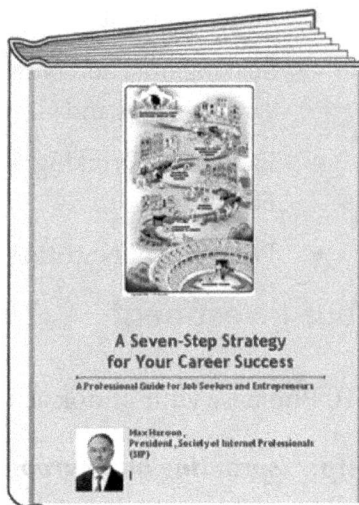

A Seven-Step Strategy
for Your Career Success

A Professional Guide for Job Seekers and Entrepreneurs

Max Haroon,
President , Society of Internet Professionals
(SIP)

Your Investment

$5 Purchase your eBook at *http://career.maxharoon.org/*

Max Haroon | guide@life-transformation-institute.org

All proceed are donated to Life Transformation Institute, a non-profit, to propagate holistic education

Glossary

Allopathic - refer to mainstream medical use of pharmacologically active agents or physical interventions to treat or suppress symptoms or pathophysiologic processes of diseases or conditions. Expression is commonly used by alternative medicine practitioners.

Amalgam is an alloy of mercury with various metals used for dental fillings. It commonly consists of mercury (50%), silver (~22-32%), tin (~14%), copper (~8%), and other trace metals.

Antiseptic – to prevent infection, especially with the elimination or reduction of the growth of microorganisms that cause disease or decay.

Bacteria - are a large group of single-celled microorganisms. Bacteria are ubiquitous in every habitat on Earth, growing in soil, acidic hot springs, radioactive waste, water, and deep in the Earth's crust, as well as in organic matter and in the live bodies of plants and animals. Bacteria reproduce by splitting in two while viruses replicate themselves inside host Friendly bacteria – see Gut flora

Bacteria can be beneficial – for instance, gut bacteria help us to digest food – but some are responsible for a range of infections. These disease-causing varieties are called pathogenic bacteria.

BPA - Bisphenol A is an industrial chemical used to make polycarbonate plastic resins, epoxy resins, and other products.

Carbohydrates/Carbs – are one of three main food nutrients (protein, fat and carbs), carbs get converted into glucose (blood sugar) in our body. There are three types of carbs: Simple carbohydrates or simply bad carbs (milk, fruits and table sugar); Complex carbohydrates or simply good carbs (whole grains, vegetables, beans); fiber (psyllium, prunes).

Carcinogens - Substances and exposures that can lead to cancer are called *carcinogens*. Some carcinogens do not affect DNA directly, but lead to cancer in other ways.

Dentin (British English: **dentine**) is a calcified tissue of the body, and along with enamel, cementum, and pulp is one of the four major components of teeth. Usually, it is covered with enamel on the crown and cementum on the root and surrounds the entire pulp.

Demineralization minerals (like calcium compounds) are leached (dissolved away) from a tooth's hard tissues (enamel, dentin, cementum). In the case of teeth, demineralisation takes place as a process (over a period of time) due to the repeated exposure of a tooth's surface to acidic compounds.

Dysbiosis microbial imbalances on or within the body. Dysbiosis is most prominent in the digestive tract or on the skin, but can also occur on any exposed surface or mucous membrane.

Enzymes are living biochemical factors that activate and aid all the biological processes in the body such as digestion, nerve impulses, detoxification processes, functioning of RNA/DNA, repair and healing of the body, and even the functioning of the mind.

Essential oil - oil is "essential" in the sense that it carries a distinctive scent, or essence, of the plant. Essential oils are generally extracted by distillation. Other processes include expression, or solvent extraction. They are used in perfumes, cosmetics, soap and other products, for flavouring food and drink, and for scenting incense and household cleaning products. Essential oils are the oldest botanical medicines recorded in the history.

Food - is any substance, materials eaten, or drunk to provide nutritional support for the body or for pleasure. It usually consists of plant or animal origin that contains essential nutrients, such as carbohydrates, fats, proteins, vitamins, or minerals, and is ingested and assimilated by an organism to produce energy, stimulate growth, and maintain life.

Genetically Modified Organism (GMO) - is an organism whose genetic   material has been altered using genetic engineering techniques. Organisms that have been genetically modified include micro-organisms such as bacteria and yeast, insects, plants, fish, and mammals. GMOs are the source of genetically modified foods, and are also widely used in scientific research and to produce goods other than food.

Gingivitis - Inflammation of the gums around the roots of the teeth.

Glycemic index (GI) - is a measure of the effects of carbohydrates on blood sugar levels. Carbohydrates that break down quickly during digestion and release glucose rapidly into the bloodstream have a high GI; carbohydrates that break down more slowly, releasing glucose more gradually into the bloodstream and have a low GI.

Gums - Flesh that surrounds the roots of the teeth.

Heuristic Education relating to or using a method of teaching that encourages learners to discover solutions for themselves. Using this philosophy, what is achieved is the result of a process of trial and error (the process is not necessarily based on any set of rules).

Holistic - characterized by the view that a whole system of beliefs must be analysed rather than simply its individual components taking into account all of somebody's physical, mental, and social conditions in the treatment of illness.

Inlays - restorations that fit tightly within the tooth between the contours (called cusps). Inlays are smaller than dental crowns and onlays. Also see Tooth Restorations Insulin.

Interdental - situated between teeth.

Interproximal - between the proximal (point of contact) surfaces of adjoining teeth. Also see Interdental

Molar - adult humans have twelve molars in four groups of three at the back of the mouth. The third, rearmost molar in each group is called a wisdom tooth.

Mutagen - In genetics, a **mutagen** is a physical or chemical agent that changes the genetic material.

Neem - is a tree in the mahogany family Meliaceae. It is native to the Indian subcontinent, growing in tropical and semi-tropical regions.

Onlays - are slightly larger than regular fillings. They cover the whole chewing area and overlap the edge of the teeth so that they cover slightly the outward and inwards facing surfaces. Onlays are similar to crowns and cover more of the tooth making them more extensive in terms of coverage than inlays. Also see Tooth Restorations

Oral - belonging to the mouth including teeth, gums, and tongue.

Oral Systemic Link the link between inflammation, oxidative stress and systemic disease is an important area of interest in vascular medicine. Both the New England Journal of Medicine and the Journal of the American College of Cardiology have published papers affirming that inflammation plays a key role in the development and progression of not only coronary artery disease but also of systemic atherosclerosis. Several other studies have been published affirming the link between periodontal disease and vascular disease, including heart attack and stroke. (From dentalANTIOXIDANTS.com).

Organic food - is grown without synthetic pesticides, insecticides, herbicides, fungicides, hormones, fertilizers or other synthetic or toxic substances. No artificial flavours or colours have been added. Organic food does not include foods that have been irradiated or Genetically Modified Organisms (GMOs).

Pathogen - is a biological infectious agent that causes disease or illness to its host. It can be virus, bacteria, fungus or parasite.

Plaque – an invisible film of saliva, mucus, bacteria, and food residues that builds up (every day) on the surface of teeth and can cause gum disease (if it is not removed regularly).

Pulp - is the central part of the tooth filled with soft connective tissue. This tissue contains blood vessels and nerves that enter the tooth from a hole at the apex of the root.

Root canal – procedure is performed when the nerve of the tooth becomes infected or the pulp becomes damaged. During a root canal procedure, the nerve and pulp is removed and the inside of the tooth is cleaned and sealed.

Sanitizing - is the process of killing and/or removing bacteria and microbes with chemicals.

Scaling - removal of calculus and Plaque that attach to the tooth surfaces.

Sonic - producing sound or sound waves (also travelling at the speed of sound in air, approximately 1,220 km per hour/760 mile per hour). Dentistry uses a sonic scaling instrument for teeth cleaning. There are also many types of electric sonic brushes available for consumers.

Starch – see carbohydrates

Sterilisation - any process that eliminates or kills all forms of microbial life, using heat or chemicals.

Tooth Enamel - is the covering of a tooth. It is hardest and most highly mineralized substance of the body and is one of the four major tissues which make up the tooth, along with dentin, cementum, and dental pulp.

Toxic- containing a poison or toxin.

Virus - is submicroscopic causative agent of an infectious disease. A virus invades living cells and uses their chemical machinery to keep itself alive and to replicate itself. Examples of viral illnesses range from the common cold, herpes, hepatitis B, flu, etc. Antibiotics are useless against viral infections

Parting Gift

This is a living book,
so your comments and contributions will be highly appreciated and
acknowledged.

Send an email to book@7stepsdentalhealth.com and for your feedback,
we will send you a publication of the Life Transformation Institute as our
thank you gift.

Index

Also see Glossary of terms in previous section some of them are indexed (they are bolded)

www.ingramcontent.com/pod-product-compliance
Lightning Source LLC
Chambersburg PA
CBHW061723270326
41928CB00011B/2087